SWEET NOTHING

WHY I GAVE UP SUGAR AND HOW YOU CAN TOO

NICOLE MOWBRAY

Copyright © Nicole Mowbray 2014

The right of Nicole Mowbray to be identified as the author
of this work has been asserted in accordance with the Copyright,
Designs and Patents Act 1988.

This edition first published in Great Britain in 2014 by
Orion

an imprint of the Orion Publishing Group Ltd
Orion House, 5 Upper St Martin's Lane,
London WC2H 9EA

An Hachette UK Company

1 3 5 7 9 10 8 6 4 2

A CIP catalogue record for this book is available from the British Library.

Mass Market Paperback ISBN: 978 1 409 15484 6

Designed and typeset by Carrdesignstudio.com

Printed in Great Britain by CPI Group (UK) Ltd, Croydon CR0 4YY

The Orion Publishing Group's policy is to use papers that are natural,
renewable and recyclable and made from wood grown in sustainable forests.
The logging and manufacturing processes are expected to conform to the
environmental regulations of the country of origin.

Every effort has been made to fulfil requirements with regard to reproducing
copyright material. The author and publisher will be glad to rectify any
omissions at the earliest opportunity.

www.orionbooks.co.uk

For Mum, Dad and Natalie

ACKNOWLEDGEMENTS

Lucky I haven't got a chance of winning an Oscar, this list of thanks is pretty extreme.

There are so many people I want to thank for supporting me. Firstly, my family for putting up with me – that includes you Millie, Tilda, Ursula, Spencer. South Coast friends namely Julie and Jane and all the ex-Factory goers.

Formative years... Very grateful to Elsa, Roger, Paul; my mentors and the people that gave me the opportunity to make a living out of writing stories.

This all began at *Vogue*. Thank you Alexandra Shulman and Jo Ellison for commissioning the feature that spawned this book.

Then there's the people who helped me over these 300-odd pages: Holly Pannett, Ian Marber, Amanda Hills, Mica Engel and the Waterhouse Young team, Cecilia D'Felice, Professor Graham MacGregor, James Duigan and the Bodyism team – Lee, Becs, Tegan, Albert, Mike, Tom, Toby and the rest of you guys – thanks for all the squats and shakes.

To everyone at the *Guardian Weekend* Magazine who put up with me while writing this – Clare, Melissa, Ruth, Nina, Simon, Bim...

Jane Sturrock, Emma Smith, Jon Elek, Jessica Gulliver and the people at Orion and United Agents who persuaded me it was possible to do Sweet Nothing in six weeks. And Rowan Lawton. I owe you one.

And all my sweet buds – it's all because of you. Nicole and Nick, Nell and Will, Gemma and Stark, Bobby and Helena, Maya, all the Kates, Olivia, Tracey, Emma, Sarah, Sam, Katy, Kevin, Cosmo, Mia, Aspen and all of the people I have forgotten. You rule.

CONTENTS

INTRODUCTION

'It ain't the fat, people, it ain't the fat'
Professor Robert Lustig, *The Bitter Truth*

What would you say if I were to let you into a little-known way to quickly and easily make yourself look younger and thinner? There are side effects though: you'll feel more happy and confident, your sleep will improve and you'll no longer endure cravings for junk food.

Best of all, this change requires no financial investment, no pills and no expensive doctors.

Are you interested?

Okay, well, it's simple. All you have to do is cut down on the amount of sugar you eat.

It may sound miraculous, but all of these things have happened to me in the two years that I've been off the white stuff. In 2012, I ate granola, sushi and sweets and drank sugary drinks such as cocktails, fresh juices and smoothies on a regular basis. I thought I was having the time of my life. The only downside was, at a size 16, I was two or three dress sizes bigger than I am now, which often made me glum. Don't misunderstand me, there's nothing wrong with being a size 16 – we all know it's the average dress size for a woman in the UK – but I didn't really understand why I couldn't drop inches. Sure I had a 'sweet tooth', but I exercised, I didn't eat lots of crisps or fried foods, I never had rich or oily meals. What was going on? I thought that it was saturated fat that was bad for you, and that you could burn off the sugars you consumed if you were an active person, as I was.

Not so.

Eating a diet high in sugar wasn't only wrecking my dreams of an hourglass figure. What I hadn't twigged, back in the spring of 2012, was that what I was eating was also causing the fast-growing crop of fine lines on my face that I was accumulating in what seemed to be a very short period of time. Despite having never suffered with my skin before, in my late twenties and early thirties I'd begun suffering with acne and pigmentation. Aside from these visible changes, I was increasingly snappy, dogged by mood swings that would make me the life and soul of the party one minute, then grumpy, angry and upset the next. Although I have always been quite a sensitive soul, in my bad moods I never felt far away from dissolving into tears at the slightest provocation.

I put these mood swings down to the fact that I was tired.

Although I got off to sleep without any problem, I'd frequently wake in the middle of the night and sometimes stay awake for a couple of hours before managing to drop off just before I needed to get up in the morning.

Back then, it never dawned on me that my food intake had anything to do with all of this, or with the fact that my hormones were up the creek and I suffered painful irregular periods. I knew my weight was directly related to what I was eating, but those other symptoms... they couldn't be to do with what I was eating, could they?

Of course they could; and indeed, they were. I know this because in June 2012, I cut the majority of sugar out of my diet and, within a matter of months, all of these things had remedied themselves.

I'm an unlikely pin-up for a healthy lifestyle. Throughout my teens and twenties I would have been the first at the bar after work ordering a bottle of nice white wine or a double gin and tonic. I've never been good on detoxes, juice cleanses or fad diets – although I have tried to cut out both bread and cheese before, with limited success. I also experimented with the Dukan Diet and managed to stay on it for about two weeks before going back to eating exactly as I had before.

In fact, I've always been rather famed for making bad decisions. At nine I decided to flush my sister's beanbag frog down the loo. It was a smart move, until the beans swelled up and blocked the whole toilet. At 16 I decided to get a tattoo on my ankle – without telling my parents – immediately before our family summer holiday. The 'it's a transfer' fib soon got found out. At age 18 I packed myself off to university in Southampton because, being from the Sussex coast, I wanted to study in a city with a beach. Little did I know – until I arrived – that the picture in the university prospectus was actually of Bournemouth, which was 30 miles away. Southampton doesn't have a beach.

But this low-sugar thing has been one of the best decisions I've made. Although it began as an experiment (a quick fix to get me in shape for summer) analysing the things I ate showed me one thing: the vast majority of my diet (including all the things I'd naively assumed were 'healthy') were actually very high in sugar. And that was before I started counting all of the things I was eating that I already knew *weren't* healthy: my afternoon chocolate fix, the occasional piece of cake, the cans of Coca-Cola when I 'needed energy'. Somewhere along the line, I'd gone very wrong.

If you're reading this book, the likelihood is, you have too. Don't feel bad, you're in good company. There are more than 1 billion overweight adults worldwide, and 300 million of them are also clinically obese. In Britain, the 2012 NHS report 'Statistics on obesity, physical activity and diet: England 2012' found that, in 2010, more than one-quarter of all adults are obese. This figure has tripled since 1980.

The NHS says added sugars can safely make up about 10 per cent of our daily calorie intake – which equals 50 g or

12½ teaspoons a day for women and 70 g or a whopping 17½ teaspoons per day for men. While they make the usual disclaimers about their figures being dependent on people's age, size and levels of activity, many researchers claim these figures should be much lower – around 6 teaspoons a day for women and 8 teaspoons for men.

However, the NHS also estimates that we're actually eating 700 g of sugar a week on average – that's a massive 175 teaspoons – and some figures claim that Britons consume an average of 238 teaspoons of sugar each week. It sounds an absurdly high figure, doesn't it? Where would you even be getting all of those teaspoons of sweetness from? Especially if you try to live a healthy lifestyle, like I did.

The answer for many of us is processed food. It's often filled with incredibly high levels of added sugar. Don't believe me? A small pot of Rachel's Organic Low-Fat Rhubarb Yogurt has 4½ teaspoons of sugar in it. Oats So Simple Apple and Blueberry Porridge has 4 teaspoons. Heinz Cream of Tomato Soup has 5 teaspoons. Half a big tin of Heinz Baked Beans has 2½ teaspoons. One Oats 'n Honey Nature Valley Granola Bar has 3 teaspoons. A 200 ml carton of pineapple juice has 6 teaspoons, and incredibly, a can of SlimFast contains 5½ teaspoons of sugar… And that's before we start on the 'treats' most of us often allow ourselves – that can of Coca-Cola gives you energy because it contains 8 teaspoons of sugar. Likewise, that delicious bag of Haribo sweets is actually just

26 teaspoons of sugar, with assorted flavourings and gelatine thrown in. While my sister Natalie and I weren't allowed to add sugar to our porridge or cornflakes while growing up, the Kellogg's Frosties we were occasionally allowed were actually 37 per cent sugar. Ouch.

I could go on, but I am sure you get the picture.

So, how did we get here? When did all this stealth sugar start finding its way into our cupboards? I asked nutritional therapist Ian Marber (a renowned nutritional therapist and author of several books about healthy eating):

'In the 1950s and 60s saturated fat came to be seen as "bad" – or fattening – because it contained nine calories per gram. At four calories per gram, carbohydrates (and sugar is a carbohydrate) began being seen as "good". The thinking was, you could eat twice as many carbohydrates as fat. Then, a landmark study in the 1970s purported to show a link between consumption of saturated fat and levels of heart disease (this has since been refuted in subsequent studies).

Nevertheless, fat began being removed from processed foods, and sugar crept in to replace it. The benefits of eating good fats were seen as irrelevant. Sugar became seen as somehow "not fattening" and fat was "fattening", because in their minds, only one thing could be.'

In retrospect, this may not have been the wisest move. Despite the British population buying fewer physical bags of sugar than ever before, we are actually consuming more of it. Coincidentally, or not, the number of obese adults is expected to double between now and 2050, going from one in four to one in two.

And you don't need to take my word for it. In the spring of this year, the UN's World Health Organization actually said that the obesity crisis was being fuelled by hidden added sugars – the likes of which I have detailed above. They want to take action and are currently considering bringing in a recommendation later in 2014 that we halve our intake of added sugars, and also reduce our consumption of sugars that are naturally present in things like honey, syrups, fruit juices and fruit concentrates.

Which is all very well, but how do we *do* it?

It's actually very easy. We just stop buying products with sugar in them. This book will tell you how to recognise products with a high level of added sugar; these can be the first things you cut out. Over the last two years, I have found it very useful to be able to put the numbers on the back of an ingredients packet into some kind of perspective. To make it easier to demystify those ingredients labels and visualise how much sugar you are eating, it may help you to know that if you divide the number of grams of sugar in an item by four, you'll get the amount in teaspoons.

Doing no more than cutting right back on your added sugars will help you to look and feel better. I went a bit further though and also limited my intake of fruit. The reason I did this was simple: I was eating so damn much of it. I'd often eat five bits a day – a fruit salad with breakfast, a banana mid-morning, some pineapple after lunch, a bunch of grapes and a satsuma or two in the afternoon – and not really move too much from my desk. I thought mainlining fruit was somehow a healthy choice and didn't know that you really don't need to eat five bits of it a day. While I may now have some dark berries with breakfast, I've incorporated many more vegetables into my diet instead. I've also tried to severely limit my intake of honey, maple syrup, agave and the like and tried to reduce the amount of high GI foods I eat, which create blood sugar spikes when we eat them – things like pasta, white rice, bread.

Don't worry if all of this sounds baffling, I'll explain the whys and hows in greater detail later on.

What I'm not going to do, however, is soft-soap you. Two years ago I was pretty ignorant about what I put into my body. The first three weeks of going cold turkey from the majority of sugar was hard and, at times, I didn't think I could do it. There were temptations and cravings. But the results were fairly instant. Within days I looked and felt healthier. Within weeks I was slimmer, with better skin and better sleep. Finally free from cravings, I felt in control of my life for the first time in a long while. Now, being low sugar is pretty easy. I'm not super thin, I'm a size 10–12, but I am a lot less wobbly. I'm fitter and my skin's clear (most of the time!). I sleep like a baby and am a nicer person to be around. I'm rarely hungry and can go out to lunch or dinner whenever and wherever I want. I don't have to count points or calories, I don't need to refer to charts. I'm not going to say I never crave a mint chocolate chip ice cream because that wouldn't be true, but I no longer feel the need to reward myself with sweet things.

And I'm not going to sit here and say that I think sugar is evil. It's not evil. Taken in moderation, it's not a poison or a toxin. A bit of it every now and then won't kill you. Consuming it in the quantities we are eating though, is a different matter altogether.

But I must caution you, I'm not an expert. I'm not a nutritionist, or a doctor or a dermatologist. I have spoken to all of those people to help you decide how to tackle your dependency on sugar – and have no doubt about it, you are dependent on it – but if you are in any doubt over whether this is the right thing for you to do, or if you are overweight, taking any form of medication or seeing your doctor for any reason, please go and speak to a medical professional before you start.

Sweet Nothing is the story of me – a normal woman in my early thirties – and my desire to find a balance between being healthy and enjoying myself. I chose to do that by quitting sugar wherever possible. The fact that you have chosen to buy this book shows that you're already one step on the road to changing your life for the better. Here goes.

Chapter One

MY HIGH-SUGAR
LIFE

'When you think about giving up,
remember why you began.'

When I was 11 years old, I was caught in the act of eating an apple crumble out of the kitchen bin. We'd all – my younger sister Natalie, then aged nine, Mum, Dad and I – been sat down at the dinner table in the dining room, enjoying a leisurely Sunday roast, but for me, the meat and veg part of the meal was the warm-up act. The main attraction of the afternoon was always Mum's homemade crumble.

Before our house was built in the 1930s, our street in Worthing, Sussex, used to be an orchard. Everyone had at least one cooking apple tree in their garden and each year, it fell to Natalie and I to trundle around the garden with some old plastic carrier bags, collecting the cooking apples from the ground, putting the rotten ones on the compost heap –

there were screams of horror if you happened to pick up one with a maggot in – and setting the rest aside to be palmed off on grandparents or friends of the family or, failing all else, eaten at every opportunity for weeks.

Unsurprisingly, crumble time came fairly regularly and it was down to my sister and I to help make the topping – no great chore bearing in mind it only consisted of butter, sugar and flour rubbed together, sometimes with a sprinkling of cinnamon added in. It was a given that Natalie and I would spend most of the time eating lumps of sugary butter – to be honest, it was the only reason either of us could be roped in to help in the first place.

There was no doubt about it, Mum's crumble was often the pièce de résistance of the Mowbray winter Sunday lunch.

So, one Sunday afternoon, when the dinner plates had been cleared and pudding time came, of course I had a helping. The topping was golden brown and toasted to perfection: crunchy, yet soft. The apple filling was peppered with raisins, cinnamon and yet more caramelised sugar. Mmmm. I poured on the custard, passed the jug on and wolfed it down.

One helping was enough for the rest of the family, but despite everyone else having stopped eating, I asked for seconds. Mum duly doled out a piffling amount. The rest of the table sat there, chatting while I stuffed my face. My parents sent over slightly disparaging looks, as if to say 'haven't you had enough yet?'.

I had not.

Two helpings down, I reached over to the dish in the centre of the table and proceeded to pick at the crumble topping. Then, Papa Mowbray cracked. I was on the receiving end of a stern telling-off, involving a table manners tirade, a sermon about eating with your fingers and some sage advice about learning when you'd had enough to eat. My grabby little sausage knuckles were metaphorically wrapped.

Yet I couldn't resist. The thought of that heavenly topping kept whirring around in my mind. Being 11 years old and having eaten a full dinner plus two helpings of dessert, I wasn't hungry. In fact, I remember feeling uncomfortably full. Yet I still wanted more. I needed to make that entire crumble mine. It was a compulsion that I couldn't ignore.

So, when the plates had been cleared away and my parents were relaxing with a glass of wine in the sitting room, I hung back in the kitchen under the guise of recording the Radio 1 Chart Show on my ghetto blaster.

Operation crumble attack had been planned like a military operation. Before anything, I needed to create a smokescreen to insure against any potential intrusions.

The customary notice was stuck onto the door: 'SHHHH EVERYONE!' it read. 'I am taping the Chart Show!'

Then came phase one: locating the delectable sugary, buttery, biscuity crumble. There was hardly any left, I knew that, but no matter.

Phase two: upon discovery, devour. It didn't take long. Mum had thrown it into the kitchen bin, assuming that I wouldn't carry on picking from it if it wasn't on the sideboard or in the fridge. She was wrong.

Undeterred, I thrust my arm in, rooted around between the vegetable peelings, located the crumble, retrieved it, sat down on the floor and proceeded to carry on where I'd left off, picking off the topping with my fingers and eating it.

Humiliatingly, that's when Dad walked in. He'd ignored the sign, ruined my recording of Black Box's 'Ride On Time' and caught me in the act. My kitchen-bin-eating shame had been made public. Even as a child, I was a fully fledged scoffer.

What happened next is best left hidden to the annuls of history, but in summary, my parents were not happy. They couldn't fathom why their daughter would rummage in the bin for food when she'd already eaten more than enough.

The answer was, of course, I was greedy. But not plain old greedy for anything. No, my insatiable appetite was solely directed at anything sweet.

Whereas Natalie was (and still is) a slender, extra-Yorkshire-pudding type of a girl, I was the chubby child who'd guzzle down all of her dinner to get to the Vienetta. Chipsticks or Monster Munch be damned, I'd choose Frosties over toast, opt for fries dunked in milkshake (don't knock it until you've tried it) instead of a burger at McDonald's and a quarter of sherbet pips from the sweet shop with my pocket money.

I divulge this rather unattractive story of gluttony for a reason. Granted, I haven't eaten out of a bin for quite some time, thankfully, but fast forward 21 years and little had changed in terms of what I actually consumed. Yes, my tastes had become a little more developed – swap the Vienetta for a blueberry and lemon millefeuille, Frosties for some granola, milkshake for a nifty mojito and sherbet pips for a large tub of sweet popcorn et voilà, you have the 32-year-old me. I'd never really worked off that childhood puppy fat either, being 5′10″, a size 14–16 and over 13 stone.

Then, on 25 June 2012 after a 6-mile cycle ride to work, I simply decided to stop eating sugar. There was no 'eureka!' moment after months of pondering, I hadn't had a close encounter with the scales (indeed I've never owned any scales), there'd been no health scare that set me off thinking I needed to change my life and I hadn't fallen under the spell of some extreme nutritionist. I'd just been feeling below par for quite some time, and, if you'll excuse the pun, I was sick of it.

I remember that day with a clarity of recollection that's probably reserved for people who are winning an Oscar or witnessing their first born get married. It was a warm, sunny Monday, the first day of the Wimbledon tennis championships and, after a rainy spring and a recent break-up I decided I wanted to get some fresh air before the doubtlessly long work day ahead. I dusted off my ever-so-pretentious Pashley bicycle to journey from my one-bedroom loft apartment in Brixton, south London, to the newspaper office where I worked, in Kensington, west London.

As I slowly cycled through Battersea Park and over the Albert Bridge across the Thames, I pondered why I'd been feeling so sluggish. I'd been so concerned about my ongoing tiredness that I'd recently bought a carbon monoxide detector to see if I was being secretly poisoned in my flat. It was the only thing I could think of to cause such a feeling of malaise. I wasn't being poisoned, so the mystery continued.

I felt that my life, and my health, was spiralling out of control. I was newly single and unhappy with many elements of my career, but that doesn't explain why an average, healthy young woman – who takes pricey vitamins by the handful, eats high-quality food and exercises – would suffer ten bad bouts of tonsillitis in two and a bit years. Why, when I'd been going to the gym and seeing a personal trainer, I was still overweight? Why I was sleeping poorly, waking up in the night, then struggling to get back to sleep? Despite having great skin as a teenager, I'd started to suffer sporadic outbreaks of acne over the past few years, which no amount of care, expensive skincare or intense facials were helping. My fine lines and open pores – both telltale signs of prematurely ageing skin – were becoming quite noticeable. My periods were out of control – irregular and painful. I had dark shadows under my bleary eyes and woke up in the morning fantasising about eating a packet of chocolate biscuits. The cravings would stay most of the day and the prospect of not having a treat made me feel grumpy and cross. How had this happened?

I was puzzled. Nothing made sense to my foggy brain. So, I did what I always did in those situations. I focused on giving myself a treat because I was doing something virtuous. In my mind, cycling to work that morning meant that, like most other mornings, I could treat myself to what I considered to be a healthy Granola Parfait from Le Pain Quotidien. Le Pain is a chain of posh Belgian cafés that are slowly colonising London and New York and it has an outpost right opposite the entrance to my office. Most mornings at about 10 a.m. you would find me heading straight for it. This morning was to be no different.

I know the majority of you will be unaware of what a Granola Parfait is, so let me initiate you. A Granola Parfait goes something like this: a large-sized plastic shaker beaker consisting of one-third low-fat plain yoghurt, one-third granola (a baked muesli mix often sweetened with honey, agave or sugar, containing oats, nuts, seeds and dried fruit), and one-third fruit salad.

Alongside my granola, I'd normally order a large fresh orange juice. Mmmm, I thought, that's tasty and healthy. In fact, it's probably two of my 'five a day' right off the bat.

So, that was breakfast taken care of, and as I cycled on, I began to consider what I would be having for lunch. Oooh, I remembered, lunch was a trip to the sushi place with my colleague Olivia. It was something that we did quite regularly but I always looked forward to actually getting away from my desk for the 30 minutes it took to walk to the place and back again – it certainly beat eating lunch at my desk.

By the time I got home later, I reasoned, I'd probably just make a bowl of pasta or something as a quick meal before crashing into bed as I had a longstanding arrangement that couldn't be cancelled to meet a contact for cocktails at a new speakeasy-style bar that had just opened. Nevertheless, as I approached work, I was glad to have at least one thing sorted for the day – my food itinerary was in order.

Then, just as I was parting with the £6 for breakfast (I know, extortion) the penny dropped. With the greatest respect to Le Pain Quotidien (who also make lots of nice healthy things like super-grain quinoa salads), I deduced that a Granola Parfait probably contains a hell-load of sugar and isn't intended to be eaten every single day. Then there's the OJ. My close, and very slender, friend Jane had maintained for years that fruit juice was the devil's drink, saying 'it contains all the sugar of fruit and none of the good pulp and fibre'.

Suddenly, I got the fear. My pricey breakfast choices were probably a lot less virtuous than I'd previously figured.

Traipsing into the office with my parfait-juice combo in hand, I considered my lunch plans. A blow-out breakfast isn't so bad as long as lunch is healthy, is it? Sushi – favourite food of the supermodels and celebs the world over – has got to be good for you.

A quick internet search revealed that while it is low in saturated fat, sushi was most certainly not the slenderising lunch I'd imagined it to be for all these years. The fish part is great (and it's tiny, how bad could that bit be?), but the white rice – a refined carbohydrate that turns to sugar in the body – is also often marinated in sugar and a sweet rice wine sauce called mirin to make it sticky and give it that distinct sushi rice flavour. In fact, some people call nigiri – the little rectangles of rice with fish on the top, my lunchtime staple – a 'sugar bomb'.

So wait, what?

My 'healthy' breakfast was sugar filled? I'd often snack on a banana or a handful of raisins (sugary) or other dried fruit (ditto) at my desk before my lunch, which was also, I now knew, high in sugar. My lunch wasn't ideal and my snacks were always all sweet. I hardly ate any protein at all most days. In an instant, my world shifted on its axis.

I suppose I'd always naively assumed that as I didn't add sugar to anything and wasn't eating very much saturated fat that I was somehow eating healthily. I lived my life at a frenetic high-stressed pace and depended upon quick nutritious foods that would keep me going.

The rest of my diet followed the same pattern. Although I wouldn't contemplate having a burger, a pizza or fish and chips for lunch (far too fattening), I would happily have something containing quite a lot of white rice, a chocolate bar or a little cake a few hours later, some grapes, pineapple or some dried mango and a can of Diet Coke (or sometimes real Coke if it was a horrendously hard day) at 4 p.m. I'd graze throughout the day and into the evening on a never-ending supply of tangerines or grapes. Forget 'five a day', I was getting about ten, and almost all from fruit.

My job had meant I'd become stuck in a stressful long-hours culture. An early finish would mean getting home at 8 p.m. and while I never gave in to the temptation of the microwave meal – because I've always refused to have a microwave – I often had a 'healthy' stir-fry with a sweet chilli sauce and white rice, or pasta of some kind, before collapsing onto the sofa with a glass of red wine.

That was a good day.

However, it was not uncommon to leave the office at 10 p.m. after a 12-hour slog with no real break. As I'd have been flat out all day, chances are the shops were shut and there was nothing much in the fridge. In which case, after a taxi ride home, dinner would be whatever I had in the freezer – namely half a tub of Ben & Jerry's Cookie Dough ice cream (of which I ensured there was always a ready supply) – and a glass of red wine.

While I didn't splash out on takeaways too often, because I, hilariously, thought them to be unhealthy, when I did, I'd go for Thai. So, I looked it up, that morning of 25 June. Thai food is one of the sweetest cuisines you can eat – sweet chilli dip is one of the more obvious examples, but less visibly, palm sugar is often added to sauces and curries. I'd never countenanced it before.

I love hanging out with my friends, and am fortunate enough to have made a lot of very good ones. But what was our number one hobby? Going out for dinner, cocktails and chat. 'Bartender?! Mine's a piña colada. Oh, wait…'

I was dumbstruck. While I'd long nursed a love affair with food, it was becoming patently apparent that, as so often in my romantic life, I'd fallen for a wrong'un. My partnership with food was one that took a lot but gave nothing in return. Indeed, nutritionists believe refined sugars – ones that aren't naturally occurring in fruit, vegetables, dairy products, etc. – to be a nutritional desert. While refined sugars may provide short-term readily available energy that we measure in terms of calories, they bring no other nutritional benefits at all. They're empty. They give nothing to the body. And many also claim that, despite what the multi-billion pound food industry wants us to believe, the body does not require any carbohydrate from added sugar for energy. In other words, my thinking that I 'needed' a chocolate bar or a fruit smoothie or a huge banana before I clambered on my bike to cycle home was not strictly accurate.

As I sat on the internet that June morning I learnt that most nutritionists agree that refined sugar is completely unnecessary in our diets. Yet, if I were to eliminate every sweet thing from my diet, it wouldn't leave me with very much.

I was mystified. Before that morning, I thought I ate a balanced diet. In fact, I'd go so far as to say I considered it healthy. I always got my much-fabled 'five a day'. I drank lots of water and wouldn't dream of ordering a bacon sandwich at the canteen for breakfast, or wolfing down a pain au chocolat on the way into work. I'd always go for a dish that came with rice over something that came with chips, never ate anything fried and tried to eat as little meat as possible. This was partly because at the age of 27, I'd been diagnosed with something called 'hypertrophic cardiomyopathy' – a genetic heart condition, which is related to Sudden Adult Death Syndrome (also known as Sudden Arrhythmic Death Syndrome).

While I had no symptoms and was not thought to be at risk from the severe forms of the condition, living with a heart condition so young was a terrifying prospect. The disease meant that my heart muscle was thickened in places and therefore I'd have to take a beta blocker every day for the foreseeable future, the aim being to make my heart work less hard.

Although I've never been a massive drinker, I cut down overnight. Moderate boozing (not easy for a journalist), low-fat food and plentiful exercise became my mantra. But no matter how much I exercised or how hard I tried, I couldn't seem to shift a stubborn couple of stone that resolutely clung to my tummy and sides. Without any medical basis, I self-diagnosed the beta blockers as being responsible in some way; perhaps they slowed down my metabolism. While my arms and legs were pretty slim I, mysteriously, had a fat back. You know, that area under your bra strap that you can sometimes catch in one of those horrible reverse-view changing room mirrors? Ugh. My tummy wasn't big and round, but I had one too many rolls when I sat down – and maybe when I stood up too. Try as I might, there was no shifting it. It was as if the extra weight were superglued on.

Although my weight has never been a big deal to me (or my boyfriends), and I've never been aware of being subjected to mean comments – my podgy tummy had started to make me feel less confident. But, as every balanced individual knows, there's more to life than appearance and on top of how I looked, I just didn't feel well.

So, I decided, right there and then, sat at my desk on the morning of 25 June 2012, that I was going to ditch the sugar. I wanted to make a change for my health, not just my waistline. And here's why. I hate diets. Not only do I loathe the idea of all those charts and restrictions about what you are allowed on one day and what you're not the next, I've long been of the belief – formed after watching people follow programmes such as Slimming World, Weight Watchers and LighterLife to no avail – that they often don't work in the long-term. I know they have many success stories and I'm not saying there's anything wrong with the regimes themselves, but I do believe they are almost impossible for many people to actually live with forever. 'Dieting' often makes people feel miserable and imposes ridiculous rules on them that they can't possibly adhere to for long. A weight-loss plan that tells you to eat potatoes, pasta and sandwiches and encourages you to fill your drinks with artificial sweeteners and indulge in a glass of wine when you like – all strategies that run directly counter to the advice of most dieticians – is probably not going to equip you with the strategies you need to maintain a healthy weight for the rest of your life. It's long been my opinion that a plan that categorises foods as 'sins' but allows you to eat a certain amount per day isn't creating either a healthy attitude towards food or a model for sustainable weight loss.

Ditching much of my sugar intake, I thought, was one thing I could do, wherever I was and whoever I was with. There are no traffic lights, no points systems, no calorie counting. The rules are simple:

- ◆ No alcohol (gulp)
- ◆ No processed food – cakes, bread, sweets, biscuits, ice cream, puddings, sauces and the like
- ◆ No artificial sweeteners (one, called Neotame, has been found by researchers at Harvard University to be between 7000 and 13,000 times sweeter than sugar), which wreck the palate and create cravings for the real thing
- ◆ Severely limited amount of fruit

Instead I'd get my nutrients from upping my vegetables and, wherever possible, I'd try to avoid refined carbohydrates

– pasta, bread, white rice, refined cereals and potatoes – all foods that have a high GI (in other words, they score highly on the Glycaemic Index – a scoring system to show how quickly something releases its sugars into the body). Eating these foods causes your body to release a surge of insulin that converts the sugars you're consuming into stored fat. It's not good for the body, the brain or the waistline.

The magnitude of my impending life change was not lost on me. I'd always envisaged myself to be more Nigella Lawson than Gillian McKeith and ditching sugar and all the fun that goes with it would mean immediately changing my whole life – not just what I put in my mouth. I really hated the feeling of being hungry, it made me miserable and I fully expected to be feeling this way fairly often, bearing in mind most of the things I ate were about to be excised.

I fretted about my social life, too. Would it survive? My friends were all like me: not faddy eaters but fun, happy-go-lucky carefree young women who were not hung up on food, at least not as far as I was aware. I really didn't want to become that neurotic girl who eats before she goes to a restaurant and then pretends she's not hungry because there's nothing on the menu she can eat (this really happens in London, and quite often).

Cooking dinner too… Could I make that fun without desserts? I love to bake and enjoy looking after people – a batch of my light-as-air chocolate brownies could remedy almost any ill. What about other people's dinner parties? How would I fare at making chit-chat with people I don't know if I couldn't indulge in a couple of glasses of booze and a dessert?

Then there's romance. I mean, how would that work? I could never have contemplated jettisoning sugar while I was in a relationship with the last man I'd been dating. Indeed, if you thought my sugar intake was bad, wait until you hear his. Always the life and soul of the party, this man – let's call him Chris – knew exactly how to bring out the bon viveur in me. We'd regularly stay out until 3 a.m. drinking cocktails, then, on the way home he'd ask the taxi to wait while he went in to a 24-hour shop to buy bags of sweets and cans of fizzy drinks. His idea of a quiet night was to go to the cinema and order a giant tub of sweet popcorn and a sharing bag of chocolates that would then be tipped into the bucket as a kind-of sugary lucky dip. It was the stuff dentists' nightmares are made of, and I loved it.

But Chris was gone (more on that later), and those other doubts? Well, rather than bombarding myself with negative thoughts, I decided to park them and instead deal with them as and when they arose. The last thing I needed was to focus on the negatives and so, instead, I began planning which size 14 white swimsuit I would buy (the 'in' thing in the summer of 2012) for a forthcoming trip to Spain with a friend. I had seven weeks to get myself in shape to wear it.

I'm a fairly strong person with oodles of willpower, but I knew I wouldn't be able to do this on my own. I'd need support.

But, somehow, I couldn't imagine many people from my group of party-going 30-something friends being massively enthused by a pact to stop drinking. Eating oatcakes instead of Hotel Chocolat's salted caramel puddles in the afternoon would probably not go down too well either.

So, instead, I went online and bought a copy of James Duigan's *Clean and Lean Diet* book – a tome that I hoped was to become the roadmap to guide me to the new, healthy me. It arrived the next morning before I left for work. I opened it and read the following words:

> 'First off, it's important to understand that your weight and health are not separate issues,'... 'Being overweight is a symptom of being unhealthy... You must believe you can do this. It doesn't matter how often you have failed in the past – your past does not equal your future. What matters now is focussing on what you want, identifying what you need to do to get it and taking consistent action. Your health and happiness are important so stand strong.'

So, stand strong is what I would do. James' regime has a 14-day 'kickstart' plan, which is pretty strict yet do-able. There were no punitive measures for faltering, simply pick yourself up, dust yourself off and get on with the plan. I'd made up my mind. I was going to do it, go cold turkey from all the foods

I thought I enjoyed. I wasn't sure how long I would be able to stick at it – my attempt at the high-protein Dukan Diet didn't last long. But I felt differently about going low sugar. I wanted to give it my best shot, not least because many of the maladies I'd been noticing in myself – everything from wrinkles to a fat back and belly to mood swings and lethargy – were written there in black and white as symptoms of an over-consumption of sugar. I had to change.

So that morning, before work, I threw all the obvious signs of sugar out of my cupboards. My sugary food filled three black bin liners. Four different half-used varieties of honey, including a very pricey one from Hawaii that tasted like fudge, all binned. My favourite cordials – elderflower, ginger and lemongrass – poured down the sink, alongside the large cartons of fruit smoothies I'd slug as a pre-breakfast snack before I made my way to work. All stir-in sauces, dips and ketchups were thrown away. Cereals, pasta, rice, bars of dark chocolate, biscuits, beers and booze were placed outside the door of my lovely supportive neighbour and fellow sugar fiend, Sam, a 6′ 4″ inch rugby player who I knew would make light work of them.

Lastly, I tackled the beloved freezer. Three pristine tubs of Ben & Jerry's were taken out to the wheelie bin in the front garden in preparation for the bin men's imminent arrival.

And that was it. I went back upstairs, stood back and surveyed the cupboards. They were almost completely bare. There was no going back.

Plus, there was no way I was ever going to be able to live a completely 'sugar-free' life. No one can, it's virtually impossible. Sugar is a form of carbohydrate and is present, to varying degrees, in naturally occurring unprocessed nutritious foods, such as dairy products (milk, cheese) and vegetables, including super-healthy greens such as spinach, kale and cabbage. It's in whole grains (brown rice, spelt, quinoa) and nuts. I had to come to find my own version of a sugar-free lifestyle, one that would enable me to be me, just a less sugar-coated version of me.

I felt both exhilarated and excited, depressed and daunted. I wondered how I would mark the day without my 'treat milestones': the getting-to-work granola, the post-meeting banana, the post-lunch pineapple, the pre-meeting chocolate bar, the pre-cycle can of Coke... Enough already! I clambered on my bicycle and cycled to work.

That first day passed uneventfully, and I only remember what happened because I wrote it in my copy of the *Clean and Lean Diet* book. I had eggs from the canteen for breakfast, with some grilled mushrooms and a cup of good-quality coffee. Lunch was a hearty dressing-free pick-and-mix salad from a large healthfood shop called Whole Foods Market, conveniently located beneath the building I worked in. By the afternoon I was 'hangry' – what my friends and I call the feeling of being hungry and angry at the same time – but instead of sweets I snacked on a couple of oatcakes with some hummus. Dinner?

Grilled chicken, sliced avocado and a spinach, rocket and watercress salad with a touch of olive oil. I ate a small pot of plain full-fat Greek yoghurt for pudding with a few toasted flaked almonds and some cinnamon sprinkled over the top, washed down with water and went to bed at 9.30 p.m. Day one had been a success.

Day two, however, was anything but a breeze. Overnight, apparently, someone had removed my brain and filled the space it had previously occupied with a pile of very jangly, piercing shrapnel. Moving my head from side to side as if I were saying 'no', produced such an acute pain it made me want to vomit.

It was interesting to find that nixing sugar – an ingredient many claim is not addictive – created this intense physical reaction in me. I struggled through work, drinking as much water as I could handle, yet feeling progressively worse. It was as if I were coming down with the flu. My limbs ached and I felt wretched. I had to leave my bike at work and take a taxi home. I hobbled out to the waiting car, bent over like a very elderly lady. I wobbled up the two flights of stairs to my loft, fantasising about my jumbo sofa that was waiting for me up there and duly plonked myself flat, staring up at the ceiling in complete agony.

For the entire day, a searing thudding had occupied my every waking minute, but now it felt as if my eyes had stopped working. I felt like they couldn't focus, the television seemed blurry and, unfortunately, whoever had replaced my brain with shrapnel had also stuck sandpaper to the backs of my eyelids, meaning every time I shut my eyes to blink, a horrendous scratchy sensation shrieked through me. I felt so weak and ill, I genuinely thought I'd been poisoned. Either that, or I was very sick.

I endlessly fantasised about a can of full-sugar Coca-Cola and a tube of Smarties. The thoughts whirred round and round my head on a loop. There was only one thing for it. I had to have some sugar to see if what I was feeling was withdrawal or something more serious.

I – again – rummaged in the bin to dig out the bottle of lemongrass and ginger cordial that I'd unceremoniously dumped into the recycling box the day before. There was a trickle left and I duly poured it into a small glass, topped it up with water and lay back on the sofa to slurp it down in front of the Wimbledon highlights. Within minutes my headache had gone. I felt energised, happy – and horror-struck. Those god-awful feelings I'd been getting weren't me coming down with some grotesque summer flu. I was withdrawing from the sugar and it looked like it was going to be worse than I'd imagined.

I'd be lying if I said I didn't consider giving up there and then. I pondered that instead of going cold turkey, I could perhaps just cut down? Swap some things and keep others. But deep down I knew. I knew I wouldn't be able to kick my addiction – and while professional opinion is divided, an addiction is how I now saw it – in that way. In his book, James

Duigan advises people that they 'don't have to stick to every rule religiously', which is doubtless sage advice. But I knew what I was like. If I allowed wriggle room – a smoothie in the morning, cakes on special occasions – I would gradually slip back into my dependency on the substance my dad has long called 'white poison'. The past two days had shown me more than ever that I needed to quit. And now.

By the time I clambered into bed at 10 p.m., that small cordial sugar hit had almost worked its way out of my system. The headache was back and I felt quite weak. I got between the sheets but couldn't sleep. The time ticked on: 11 p.m., midnight, 1 a.m., 2 a.m. all passed without any sign of the land of nod. I felt wired and exhausted at the same time. Happy days.

Instead of concentrating on how bad I felt, I decided to look at the benefits. I was never going to have to go through Detox Day Two again, which felt like an overwhelming positive. I was 48 hours into the healthier, slimmer, less food-obsessed me. I couldn't wait to stop having energy peaks and troughs and, instead, cruise through each day on a level playing field, free from cravings and strange compulsions to eat badly. I would find a new way to 'reward' myself after a hard day, or a difficult conversation or an exercise session, perhaps with something that doesn't make you fat, ill and prematurely aged in the way that excess sugar does.

While the vast majority of doctors, nutritionists, cardiologists, oncologists, immunologists, endocrinologists (diabetes and hormone specialists) and more all agree that the Western populace eat too much sugar and reducing your sugar intake will benefit your health, I knew that I needed to find a balance between enjoying life and living healthily. But could I find it?

All of these short-term feelings would be worth it, ten-fold, when I could meet someone new without worrying they'd notice all my spots before they noticed anything else about me. When I could wear a pair of denim cut-offs feeling self concious about my wobbly thighs. I couldn't wait to feel confident in my cozzy on the beach later that summer.

In desperation, I did what any 21st-century person does when they need support. I turned to social media. On the 26 June 2012, I wrote this:

'Trying to give up sugar. Two days in and I have the most banging headache – and 12 more days to go. Watch out world… Grouchy.'

My wonderful friends wrote messages of support underneath. 'Best thing you'll ever do, good luck' wrote Ali. And Bruno 'You can do it! I'm trying to cut down and I do feel better just having less anyway.' 'It's basically living hell for four days but the serene, smug satisfaction of doing it for a few weeks is worth it (not to mention having lovely glowing skin)…' wrote Martha. And then there was Jill. 'Oooh I did it about three years ago,' she wrote, 'and only lasted two days. It was as if someone was playing Jedward on a loop inside my brain. Horrible.'

I had been warned.

Chapter Two

EARLY DAYS

I tried to put Jedward out of my mind.

But the next morning my head was still pounding, possibly even more severely than the night before. It was as if my brain had dried up and was rattling around in my skull. Each time it knocked against the sides, a searing pain radiated across my forehead like someone was making me wear a sweatband of barbed wire. Not nice.

The situation was not aided by the fact that I'd only descended into a fitful, clammy sleep at 4 a.m., after lying in bed feeling sick for six hours. Then, four hours after I'd finally arrived in the land of nod, I had to drag myself out of bed to start my Thursday.

I needed to remind myself why I was doing this and so I decided to make a list to put on my fridge for whenever I was feeling down in the dumps or liable to go and wolf down a tub of ice cream – which at the moment was pretty often. Nutritional therapist Ian Marber will go into the biochemical reasons for giving up sugar in more detail later in the book, but to tide you over, here's an exact copy of the note I had pinned to my (treat-free and sadly empty) refrigerator:

◆ **Treat your ticker nicely!**

Excess sugar consumption is linked to obesity, which is linked to heart disease and can affect the pumping mechanism of your heart. You've only got one and you need it, so it's probably something you should look after.

◆ **Help your hormones and lower your risk of cancer**

Eating too much sugar can cause the body to become insulin resistant. Studies have shown that people who are insulin resistant are more susceptible to cancer.

◆ **Love your liver**

Studies have shown that a diet high in sugar causes similar damage to that done by heavy drinking.

◆ **Lose your love handles**

Eating too much sugar makes you fat; this is something everyone agrees on. And being overweight can lead to serious health issues like diabetes, which has its own problems.

◆ **Avoid premature ageing**

So, what would you rather have – a chocolate bar or deeper crow's feet at the age of 40?

◆ **Revisit the land of nod**

What you wouldn't give for a night of unbroken sleep? How about not having that can of fizzy drink and stepping away from the chocolate? Because it's as simple as that.

I did not feel at all well. But, to be honest, this was something I had expected. While some experts say that sugar is not addictive, a quick Google search of the words 'withdrawal symptoms sugar' reveals what anyone who has ever tried to kick the habit knows. Sugar withdrawal is a serious business. If you've previously had a high sugar intake, as I had, giving it up is described in various places online as both painful and debilitating.

I knew I was dependent on sugar. Properly, hopelessly, chemically and emotionally dependent on it. Sweet things – not only the obvious culprits (fizzy pop, bags of jelly sweets or chocolate bars), but also carbohydrate-dense and processed foods, especially foods with a high GI (Glycaemic Index), such as white bread and white rice – were on my mind almost all of the time. It was as if I were in love with them. Aside from the physical withdrawal symptoms of addiction that I (and my poor friends and colleagues) was going to experience in the coming days and weeks – shakes, weakness, nausea, spots, lethargy, headaches, irritability – I spent hours and days thinking about foods I was trying not to eat. Don't panic. This didn't last long, but it did feel bizarre. I'd never really given my sugar consumption much conscious thought before, perhaps because I'd often pre-empted cravings or obsessive thoughts about sweet things by acting on them before it got to that stage.

This phenomenon is not, however, uncommon. Research last year using brain scans at the New Balance Foundation

Obesity Prevention Center in Boston has shown that sugary foods could be physically addictive and stimulate cravings in much the same way as an illicit drug, which could go some way to explaining how I'd got trapped in a cycle of eating them. Plus, of course, I really liked the taste of them.

Now, if you are trying to give up sugar, or considering it, I realise my testimony may be causing you to have a rethink. But the whole 'secret' to giving up sugar is to change the focus of your rewards from the short term to the long. I had to remember that although I felt like I was somehow being hard done-by by not having a biscuit when they were being offered around the department at work, my reward was actually going to come two months down the line when I was one dress size (maybe more) smaller than I was that day. I tried to focus, too, on the fact that, within days, I would be feeling better than I had in months and that would only continue to improve. What I didn't understand at the time was why I was feeling this way. I have since asked Ian Marber, a nutritional therapist, why I felt the withdrawal so keenly.

'Anyone quitting sugar would experience some feelings of withdrawal,' he says. 'In your case, I would imagine your blood glucose levels would have been out, your protein levels were potentially low and your adrenal glands would have been working quite hard – this explains those feelings of extreme highs and lows. Excessive sugar intake depletes the body's store of B-vitamins [they are partially responsible for getting energy from food and maintaining healthy brain functioning and mental clarity] so that would explain the feelings of mental fogginess that's often experienced by people quitting sugar.

'Another contributing factor is that people who eat a high-sugar diet often have bacteria that thrive on sugar living in their gut. When you cut off the food source, the bacteria start shouting "feed me!", which often contributes to feelings of fatigue.'

So far, so gross. 'You can also think of it like this,' Ian says. 'Giving up sugar is like changing fuel tanks. Sugar is an incredibly available source of fuel for the body. Take that away and your system has to work harder to get energy from the next source of fuel, which is complex carbohydrates (wholegrain breads, pulses, starchy vegetables). Take those away – or reduce them as many people do when they are trying to quit sugar – and you've now got to dig down deep into your fat stores for energy, which is like trying to get into your deposit account when you've already shown your bank manager that you're a nightmare with money.'

So what was I missing the most? Breakfast. Undoubtedly my beloved breakfast.

Orlando, Florida, 1992. A tubby 13-year-old me with a permed bob (including the fringe), a new pair of hi-top LA Gear trainers and an oversized Esprit T-shirt, first tasted waffles with maple syrup in a Denny's restaurant. It was life-changing. I would have eaten that breakfast every day for three weeks had my parents let me. At that age, waffles with maple syrup would have been my death row meal – had I known what that was. I'd happily have eaten it each and every time I sat down at the table.

Of course, as soon as I became image conscious and realised the link between things like waffles at every meal and my expanding waistline, I quit choosing that type of thing for breakfast when faced with it on a menu. One thing that hasn't changed though is my long-standing belief in the merits of starting the day with a hearty breakfast – one that's eaten sitting down, accompanied by tea and the trimmings. Not for me was this guzzling a croissant out of a greaseproof bag on the way to work routine, or wolfing down one of those measly 'breakfast bars', which look about as filling as a piece of paper.

Yet this sugar purge made me think: why do the majority of us in the Western world rarely eat savoury food at breakfast? Because, although I quickly ditched my burgeoning waffle dependency, I must confess to throwing away no fewer than four different sugary breakfast cereals during my cupboard mine-sweep. There was an expensive 'artisan' granola, a box of Dorset Cereals high-fibre muesli, packed to the rafters with juicy dried fruit, some good old-fashioned Kellogg's Frosties and a box of Fruit and Fibre. Binning those left me feeling like I had few culinary options when I managed to drag myself out of bed in the morning. It seemed that things that aren't processed and packed full of sugar involve more effort – and time – than simply tipping a packet into a bowl in the morning.

In fact, in my diary entry for day three of my sugar detox I wrote. 'Breakfast came and went without occasion. Ate a piece of steamed salmon and some green beans. It didn't put a spring in my step. Ugh. Can't wait for lunch – it's more of the same. Oh sorry, I CAN.'

So, come on, aside from eggs or something like a full English breakfast over the weekend, when was the last time you started the day with something savoury? The body converts wheat to sugar faster than any other grain – rice, barley or oats, for example – so if you said toast, that's a bad start (plus bread often has sugar added into it anyhow). Then let's consider the fact that few of us eat our toast plain, as in without jam, honey or any other sweet spread. I'd wager hardly any of us wolf down unadulterated porridge with no sugar, jam, banana or honey, unless our cupboards are bare. Even plain cornflakes (which many of us load up with sugar) already have sugar added to them in the manufacturing process.

And breakfast was my big thing. I could eat a mountain of granola or fruit muesli with a fruit yoghurt and often with fresh fruit on top. Were I to have porridge, it was unfailingly topped with both banana and honey. All washed down with copious amounts of fresh (the 'healthy' stuff, not that crap from concentrate) orange juice. Were I out for a work breakfast at somewhere posh – which was happening about twice a week – I'd opt for a fresh pineapple juice instead.

So far, so sweet.

Yet it doesn't have to be like this, indeed it isn't like this in much of the world. The Swedes and Swiss commonly eat a high-protein breakfast consisting of hard-boiled eggs, cheese, salmon and the like. The Japanese are also big on fish alongside noodles and miso soup. In India, too, breakfasts are more of a savoury affair: spicy 'beaten rice' dishes such as aval upma or nasi goreng in Indonesia.

While it's true that there aren't many of us who can face steak and eggs at 7.30 in the morning (and who wants to have to wash up all that greasy stuff before work?), it certainly feels as if our breakfasts are skewed towards sweet stuff. Can it be a coincidence, I wondered, that the countries that start their days with a giant hit of sugar, also top the obesity league tables? While there's nothing like a large bowl of sweetness to have you bounding down the garden path and on to the office, I think we all know what happens a couple of hours from then. We're hungry, grumpy and ready for a mid-morning snack.

But then, sugary cereal does have its advantages. How long do you think it takes to steam a piece of white fish? It's a heck of a lot longer than pouring some cereal out of the box I can tell you, and the house isn't left smelling too pretty.

Then there's cost. A decent box of muesli will set you back about £3.50 for what the manufacturers claim will be 18 servings (who are they kidding – 18 servings? More like six!). A small piece of fish costs just that for one day.

It's not easy to cook yourself a healthy breakfast every day. It takes effort and organisation. Rather than simply opening the cupboard, you have to use pots and pans, have all of your ingredients to hand and be prepared to clean up afterwards. I wasn't used to it. Everything felt like a lot of effort to have to make before you'd even left the house.

But I knew this was the hard bit. Because I'd told all of my family, friends and everyone on Facebook that I had ditched sugar, I couldn't crack three days in. My pride wouldn't allow it. Not to mention the fact that I'd thrown away all of my sugary food so even if I wanted something else to eat, there wasn't anything.

So, what is sugar and what was it doing to my, and your, body?

While we may not think of it in the same way as potatoes, bread and pasta, sugar is a carbohydrate. Indeed, if you are looking on food labels, you will often only see carbohydrates quantities listed, rather than sugar content.

But there are many different types of sugar and not all are created equal. Here are some of the most commonly found ones, which I have chosen to avoid if at all possible:

Refined, added or processed sugar – the type you buy in bags and add to drinks, sauces and home-baking. You know the stuff. Refined or added sugar goes by lots of different names (more on that later) and is what is also added to many convenience foods and ready meals that we buy.

Natural 'masquerading' sugars – honey, agave, maple syrup. Many people think these are much 'better' than eating granulated sugar because they are more 'natural'. We mustn't forget that granulated sugar is essentially 'natural' too, coming as it does from sugar beet or cane. Unfortunately, when we consume them, honey, agave, maple syrup and the like predominantly cause a very similar reaction inside the body – a surge in blood sugar levels – as sugar does.

Fructose – this is the sugar that comes from fruit (and also honey). While fruit has lots of health benefits and I wouldn't say it's 'bad' for you, there are plenty of other sources from which to get vitamins and fibre (like vegetables, for example). Fructose is also added to products to sweeten things, but it's different from other sugars because it's processed by the liver, not dealt with by insulin.

Simple carbohydrates – our body uses carbohydrates to make glucose. Glucose in turn gives your body energy. But carbs come in two forms. The complex ones are the good guys. These take longer to break down in the body and therefore don't create huge blood sugar spikes. Complex carbs are fibre-rich or starchy foods that haven't been refined much from their original state – things like pulses, beans, nuts, brown rice. Simple carbohydrates have a simple chemical structure – hence the name – and convert to sugar inside the body very quickly. These are less good for you. Things like white bread, white rice, cakes, crisps, sweet cereals, fizzy drinks and chocolates are simple carbohydrates. As well as causing blood sugar spikes inside the body, many of these also often contain added refined sugar, providing a horrible double whammy.

Alcohol – the fermentation process often means it's high in sugar.

Artificial sweeteners – many processed products that say they're 'sugar-free' often use synthetic sugars to create the taste of sweetness. You will recognise some of the names of these: aspartame, saccharine, sucralose, acesulfame-k, Nutrasweet, sorbitol… Some of these sweeteners are several hundred times sweeter than natural sugar. I will go into the effects of these later in the book (see page 159).

Every time you eat any type of sugar your blood-glucose level rises. How quickly depends on the type of sugar you have eaten, whether it's simple or complex, what's already in your stomach, and what you have eaten the sugar with. Ian Marber explains:

'Let's say you woke up in the morning and had a cup of tea or coffee with sugar in it, or a can of Coke,' says Ian. 'The drink has no fibre and it's got no fat, which slow down its absorption, so its journey from food to glucose in your body is as rapid as it possibly can be. This will automatically raise glucose levels in the blood. The body wants to protect itself against too much sugar in the blood, so the pancreas produces the hormone insulin, which comes along and tells the body's cells to open up to store the glucose. Insulin's main role is to manage glucose, which it does in two ways. Firstly by facilitating the entrance of glucose into the cells [to provide energy for the body], then by shovelling away the excess that can't go into the cells as glycogen [energy] stores. Once the glycogen stores are full, the body keeps the rest as fat.

'So what ingesting sugar does is firstly it triggers an insulin response, it fills your glycogen stores and gives you energy. But the downside – if there is too much – is that the effects are very temporary. It's fleeting.

Insulin, effectively, mops everything up as quickly as possible, but it doesn't leave any in reserve for later. Which explains why, an hour or so after you've eaten a meal or snack that's high in refined sugars, you are hungry again. Then you get into that spiral of thinking "what's wrong with me? I've just eaten. How can I be hungry again?".'

Eating sugar isn't a modern phenomenon. Sugar is found in the tissues of most plants and has been eaten (in its raw form as sugar cane or sugar beet) in India, Pakistan and Bangladesh since ancient times. Before long, Europeans fell in love with it, and demand in the 14th and 15th centuries meant producers were on the lookout for new lands on which to grow their crop. Plantations – many forcibly worked by African slaves – began popping up in places like Madeira and the Canary Islands, where, in 1492, sugar fell into the hands of explorer Christopher Columbus who took the treat to the New World, namely the West Indies, Cuba and Mexico, which had wetter climates better suited to growing the crop.

The horrendous history of sugar, trade and slavery is one detailed enough to have filled many books on its own, but suffice to say, once Europeans got a taste for the expensive delicacy, there was nothing we wouldn't do to get our hands on it. We colonised lands to produce it, fought the Napoleonic Wars to keep our supply routes open and even tried to grow it in dear old Blighty. The government made so much money from the taxation of it that many began calling sugar 'white gold'.

While demand was going through the roof, sugar remained a luxury until Prime Minister Gladstone abolished the substantial tax levy on sugar in 1874, putting the product within reach of the ordinary guy and gal. So-called 'white gold' ceased being so expensive and the population at large began to see the product as a necessity, rather than a luxury. Europeans fell so deeply in love with the taste of sugar that it began to be added to all manner of food and drink. And that, in a nutshell, is how our collective 'sweet tooth' was born.

Indeed, since the Second World War, food, and sugar, has been abundant for most of us in the West. The vast majority of us have never had to worry where our next meal is coming from, or been forced to go to bed hungry. We've long since stopped thinking of fruit as a 'treat'. Our taste buds have become completely accustomed to eating sugar whenever we want, in whatever we want.

Perhaps that's why many of us – myself included – often have too much of a good thing. For us, food has ceased to be fuel and become something to be fetishised. Food – and especially sweet treats – is now inherently linked to our value systems.

For example, if my boyfriend had had a crappy day at work, or if I was trying to show him just how much I loved him, I'd bake him a batch of my extra-special chocolate brownies and serve him up two, topped with vanilla ice cream. Of course, they'd be fresh out of the oven and still warm and have just the right amount of meltiness. Likewise, if he wanted an easy way to show me he loved me on Valentine's Day, when he was in my bad books (often) or for some other special occasion, I'd receive a big box of chocolates (my favourites were floral ones, like Prestat's Rose and Violet Crèmes or Rococo's Lavender Dark Chocolate).

Then there is the ultimate 'feel-good' treat: birthday cakes. I know that had someone given me a sliced avocado on oatcakes with a candle in the middle instead of a huge sugary birthday cake when I was younger, I'd probably have been a bit miffed.

Using these examples, it's easy to see how food – especially sweet food – has become loaded with meaning and emotion, and as James Duigan's *Clean and Lean Diet* book points out, it's a value system that gets put in place very young. Children's birthday parties, with their take-home bags of sweets intended to make the feel-good feeling continue just that little bit longer, are a case in point. Likewise, elaborate icing-topped birthday cakes for one-year-olds or a lollipop after you've had an injection at the doctor. It doesn't take a genius to see how we have become programmed to see food as a reward.

While there's no real problem with this if it's a once-in-a-blue-moon event – like a birthday or Christmas or some other special occasion – for many adults, treating ourselves has become a daily event. I know I saw my 4 p.m. work-day chocolate run as a 'break' from work. It was a reward for working hard and nearly getting to the end of the day. I felt I somehow 'deserved' it, especially as I'd normally have had what I thought to be a fairly virtuous lunch like sushi or a salad wrap. Were I going on a long car journey or taking a trip on a plane, I'd buy a large bag of sweets 'to keep me going'. Gym workouts would be rewarded with a freshly made big berry smoothie, because I'd 'worked so hard'… It's easy to fall into the trap.

The National Diet and Nutrition Survey – a rolling study carried out by the Department of Health and the Food Standards Agency – found that, on average, Britons eat 96.5 g of sugar per day. To make that easier for most of us to visualise, that equates to almost 24 teaspoons daily, or 168 in a week. It's a massive amount. While some of us will eat more, and some less, as the *Daily Mail* points out, 'it still means that we are getting more than the 90 g [per day] (22 teaspoons) that the UK Food Standards Agency currently says is acceptable', which to me still seems like an astoundingly high level to allow in a time when the population is getting ever fatter, but I digress.

I imagine many will be shocked at that information. I know I was. If you don't take sugar in your drinks, rarely eat cakes and otherwise live a fairly balanced existence, it's hard to imagine where that quantity of sweet stuff would come from. But, as I was learning, sugar is in virtually everything that's processed, including things that don't taste sweet. Here, in no particular order, is what I'd had to ditch after Tuesday's mine-sweep (which already felt like aeons ago):

Honey and agave I must confess, I didn't realise that natural sugars such as honey and agave (in case you are unfamiliar, it's pronounced ah-gah-vey and is made from a spiny plant native to south America) were almost as bad as refined or processed sugars. But they are. Many honeys, agaves, maple syrups and the like have been processed and remain high in calories – in fact at 60 calories per tablespoon, agave is higher in calories than refined sugar (40 calories). The idea is to use less of it, but I know I liberally poured honey into yoghurts, herbal teas and the like, imagining it to be in some way superior to other sugars. But not only are honey and its ilk implicated in weight gain, they also perpetuate the body's taste for sweet things. This is something that I hadn't really fathomed when I was so intent upon covering my organic porridge with organic honey and sliced banana throughout the winter months.

Squash, cordial and all fizzy drinks It is astounding to me that, despite their sugar content, some squashes manage to get away with claiming to be one of your 'five a day'. High in calories, low in anything else – except, for me, enjoyment – means these had to go. Although I'd always considered water something that should be somehow jazzed up, I had to accept that filling it with sugar probably wasn't a very good way of doing it.

Sauces, cook-in sauces, salad dressings, jars of things. Not only are these things heavily processed, they're almost always pretty sugary, especially the Chinese-style cook-in sauces. Binned. Here's a little known fact: many stock cubes contain sugar too. Why? I'm not sure.

Gravadlax and many cured fish. This is a shocker. Gravadlax (a cured salmon, often coated in dill) is marinated in sugar, so that's out. Likewise any honey-cured fish as well as some smoked mackerel and herring. Always check on the packet to be on the safe side.

Cakes, biscuits, sweets, chocolate, 'healthy' muesli bars. These are all highly processed with little or no nutritional value. Muesli bars are really wolves in sheep's clothing: oats, nuts and fruits stuck together in a bar by sugar. They may give you instant energy, but not long afterwards you'll crash.

Crisps. Okay, if you're going on a healthy eating kick, crisps (usually high in carbohydrates, high GI and high in fat) are one thing that probably should be cut out from the word go. While I only ate crisps once in a blue moon, it was staggering to me to find out that a small packet of those posh Sweet Chilli flavoured Kettle Chips contain 2 per cent of your daily allowance of sugar. Crisps aren't even sweet.

Anything altered to become 'low fat'. This is a big hurrah. James Duigan says to pick butter over margarine (which I've always done), regular hummus over the reduced-fat versions and the same for yoghurts. He – like many nutritionists – believes that, instead of helping you lose weight, low-fat foods actually make you fat and here are a few reasons why. Products that are modified to be low fat are often pumped full of sugar, salt and sweeteners to make up the taste. Then, because they're billed as being 'diet' foods, people believe they can eat more of them. Whereas foods with good fats in them – nuts, seeds, avocado, meat, oil, fish and seafood – keep you fuller for longer and also prompt the body to burn any fats it has stored in the cells. Good fat helps your body to absorb vitamins and minerals and it helps protect the joints. I didn't need any more reasons to ditch the Müller Light yoghurts and move on to full-fat Rachel's Organic. Skimmed milk (which has long tasted just like white water to me) was also binned in favour of semi-skimmed or whole milk.

Diet drinks containing artificial sweeteners. Think you can give up sugar and just exist on artificially sweetened things? Sorry to disappoint you. Ditching sugar also means ditching fake sugars, which, in my opinion – and that of many medical professionals – are no better for you than the real thing. While no concrete evidence has been found, there has been much debate surrounding chemical sweeteners, such as aspartame, tand the fear that they may be linked to an increased risk of cancer. Aside from this, many sweeteners are hundreds of times sweeter than natural sugar – some are even thousands of times sweeter – so consuming them isn't going to help you ignore that sweet tooth. Diet Coke and its low-calorie relatives had now been consigned to room 101.

Carbonated drinks and pop. Bad for your teeth, tummy and just about everything else. We all know fizzy pop is bad for us but most of us drink it at least a few times a week, probably because it tastes good and it's convenient. But no more. Fizzy pop has been poured down the sink.

Fruit. I know this is a controversial one and it's the main part of the sugar-free plan that my mum has long struggled to get her head around. Eating a lot of sugary fruit is not good for you. Remember when eating a piece of fruit used to be a treat at the end of a meal? While those innocent days are – for many – long gone, replaced with the likes of Häagen-Dazs and Gü chocolate puddings, it is worth remembering that fruit is incredibly high in sugar so we shouldn't be eating several pieces every day. In fact, I have learnt that most of your 'five a day' should come from vegetables rather than fruits. Thinking fruit was a healthy, low-calorie nutritious snack – and one that would help me lose weight – I had been wolfing down about five pieces of fruit every day, including many of the most sugary varieties, namely grapes, bananas, mangos, sweet cherries, apples, pineapples, pears and kiwis. So, it looked like I would be finding a new use for my fruit bowl – or just filling it with avocados, lemons and limes with the occasional helping of antioxidant-rich dark berries (here's a simple general rule to remember – the darker the fruit, the more good antioxidants it contains and, therefore, the more beneficial it is). Yet I genuinely worried about life post-pineapple. There are few things nicer than piling your plate high with sumptuous chunks of fresh pineapple when you're on holiday somewhere with a generous breakfast buffet. Still, I had to accept that until I started running ultra-marathons in my spare time – which was going to be never – my body had no use for all those sugary carbohydrates.

Dried fruit. It's probably quite an obvious one, but dried fruit is almost all sugar. Don't believe me? Take dried mango – the leathery sweet and tart strips used to be one of my favourite snacks. If you eat a 100 g serving, which is surprisingly easy to do as dried mango is quite heavy, 73 g will be pure sugar. Raisins, dates and figs aren't far behind, coming in at 65 g, 64 g and 62 g of sugar per 100 g, respectively. I had always assumed dried fruit to be relatively healthy, at least better than a chocolate bar. Bang goes another snack.

Fruit juices. A standard 330 ml serving of Tropicana contains an astounding 30 g – around 7 teaspoons – of sugar. That's almost the same as a can of full-sugar Coke. Yes, it contains vitamins and minerals but nothing that you can't get elsewhere from sources that aren't so high in sugar. One of the small bottles of Innocent Smoothies (did you know the company is now owned by Coca-Cola?) contains the equivalent of 6 teaspoons of sugar – around 26 g. While these companies are always quick to react to criticism by saying the sugars contained within these drinks are natural fruit sugars, the body reacts in a similar way to excessive amounts of fructose as it does to any other type of sugar. Lovely as they are, both fruit juices and smoothies had to go. My waistline would thank me for it, even if my desperately craving brain wasn't going to just yet.

Bread and pasta. Brits love bread. Why else would we buy 12 million loaves of it per day? I was in that number. Bread was an emotional thing for me. I've always had a special place in my heart for a nice white sandwich of the type made by my mum for my lunchbox, or a piece of doorstep white toast – so thick it had to go under the grill rather than in the toaster – liberally slathered with butter. But it had to go. I think most of us are aware that big-brand highly processed bread – the kinds that you buy in large loaves in the supermarket – often contains a lot of sugar. Partly it's a by-product of the baking process and the rest is added by manufacturers to make it taste 'better'.

But some white, brown and wholemeal loaves actually contain around 10 g of sugar per loaf and, in fact, just one slice of Kingsmill's Farmhouse loaf contains 1.8 g of sugar. Granted, that's only 2 per cent of the recommended daily intake, but many of us will have at least two slices as toast for breakfast, then two slices for lunch. Just plain, without any spreads or toppings that would equate to an astounding 8 per cent of your sugar intake. While pasta doesn't contain added sugar, the two foods are both made from highly processed wheat – a carbohydrate that's high on the Glycaemic Index and, when wheat is eaten, it converts to sugar faster than any other grain. The body then converts that sugar to fat, which is typically stored around the hips, thighs, bum and tummy. Savoury does not equal sugar free.

Potatoes. The good old floury white variety is high on the Glycaemic Index, so it had to be ditched and sweet potato eaten in its place. This one didn't strike me as a particularly great hardship as, despite being part Irish, I've never been a big spuds fan.

Alcohol. I've saved the most painful change to last, but, unfortunately booze had to go. While I knew alcohol wasn't particularly good for you, I had no concept of how sugary it really was. I have no excuse for this, seeing that I knew alcohol was made by fermenting and distilling natural starches and sugars. These sugars make it highly calorific with no nutritional value. It is what health experts would call 'empty calories'. But nutritional value or not, I'd always placed a high social value on drinking. Indeed, some of my best memories and experiences have been formed after a jar or two. Nights spent in Hawaii with old friends and new, sitting on the beach sharing bottles of Bikini Blonde beer from a local brewery. Sake-fuelled nights at karaoke bars in Tokyo. Impromptu sing-alongs to Billy Joel at a tiny jetty-side bar in Nantucket, lubricated by whisky sours. Bottles of wine at the Coach and Horses pub in Farringdon with colleagues off to dangerous far-flung places. Above all, a glass of wine in front of the telly after a long day is an instant de-stressor. I actually felt depressed just thinking about this part. While I only probably drank 12 or so units per week, they were cherished. As a single woman in her early thirties, drinking was the social glue that bound many of my friendships. What would I do with my big group of friends if we didn't go out for a drink from time to time? Should I just meet them for coffee instead? And at night? That didn't sound like fun.

Aside from these sugars, there's also sugar in milk and dairy products, vegetables, complex carbohydrates and meat, to a certain degree. I was going to keep on eating those, which is why I could never realistically say I'd gone 'sugar free'.

But it wasn't until I began clearing out those cupboards that it really dawned on me just how much my life was going to change as a result of giving up sugar. And not only recognisable sugar. Ian Marber points out that there are also the sugars we don't recognise as sugars when/if we are reading ingredients labels: sucrose, maltose, lactose, dextrose, fructose... Basically, he says, sugar is hiding in 'any ingredient ending in "-ose"'. The same goes for syrup, rice syrup, converted rice syrup, glucose syrup, cane syrup – anything that has syrup in it is also a sugar. The worst offender is high-fructose corn syrup (sometimes abbreviated to HFCS).

High-fructose corn syrup is much derided by the medical establishment. It's a cheap, highly processed man-made type of sugar that's been combined with corn syrup to form a sweetener that is easy to mix into things – fruit juices, salad dressings, baked goods. It's quickly absorbed by the liver, which turns it immediately to fat. And, as another horrible little aside, as it's man-made, your body doesn't recognise HFCS as a real food, so it never shuts off the part of your brain that controls hunger cravings. You'll just carry on eating more and more and more. Blood sugar levels rise and massive amounts of insulin are released to deal with it. This, eventually, creates that all-too-familiar 'sugar low', before the body starts feeling hungry again. All in all, a pretty horrible and pointless process.

While I knew I had to follow these guidelines as closely as I could for the first two weeks, James' book was very clear. From time to time I would make slip-ups. While I am fortunate enough to have iron willpower, I knew that staying away from drinking – or only indulging in a low-sugar drink such as vodka, soda and a squeeze of fresh lime – would be the hardest part of my new regime to stick to and I'd already made a pact that I would sometimes allow myself a glass of nice red wine when the occasion arose. But, were I to make it past the first few weeks, I'd have to accept that my holidays consisting of little more than downing a few bottles of beer on the beach every afternoon for two weeks would have to become a thing of the past. The choice was actually rather straightforward: a pint of beer can have about the same number of calories as a slice of pizza, with none of the protein, complex carbs, etc. – and I'd rather have a narrower waist than drink beer every night. For some reason, I kept lamenting the fact that I'd never been to Munich's Oktoberfest – a legendary beer festival that I've never before wanted to go to – and now there would be no point. It's strange the way your mind works when you're in withdrawal.

Talking of pizza, now's a good time to talk about my face. Spots. Lots and lots of painful spots, all of which had decided to have a party on my face within three days of me kicking sweets – as if I wasn't having a tough enough time of it already…

I've already mentioned that a large part of the reason I decided to give up sugar was because of the outbreaks of acne I'd been suffering. Although I've never thought of myself as a vain person, it turns out I am. Despite having good skin in my teens and early twenties, by the time I reached my mid-twenties, my skin had become prone to breakouts. The area around my chin and jawline was red and irritated and I'd often get big angry spots on my cheekbones. Aside from the spots themselves, the rest of my skin was very congested. I felt like it looked grey, dull and lifeless. I'd tried to modify my diet, but not in any substantial way. For example, I'd stop eating chocolate for a few weeks, see no difference, then lose the motivation and fall off the wagon. Instead of tackling the root cause of my bad skin, which it now seemed was probably too much sugar across my whole diet, I settled on having regular expensive facials. As well as the spots, I'd noticed a growing number of fine lines accumulating around my eyes and on my forehead, which I hoped facials would help. I'd also started getting pigmentation across my cheeks and on my forehead.

While my job was stressful, a big side-effect of a diet high in sugar is prematurely aged skin. Although I'll go into this further in Chapter Four (see pages 129–37), I'll let skin doctor Mica Engels of London's Waterhouse Young Clinic briefly explain what happens to your skin if you overindulge:

'There are several reasons why too much sugar is harmful for your face,' she says. 'Excessively high blood sugar causes the body to raise its production of insulin. Both of these processes cause "inflammation" in the cells, which is now thought to increase the rate at which our skin ages.

'The scientific name for this process is "glycation".
Roughly explained, excess glucose binds to the skin's
"youth proteins" – the collagen and elastin that makes
youthful complexions appear so plump and doughy –
and instead turns them brittle and stiff. The surfaces
of the cells are effectively "caramelised". Collagen and
elastin fibres in the skin can no longer perform their
most important roles – namely cell division and tissue
renewal. Without this, wrinkles and sagging skin will
appear on the face prematurely and over time, the
problem magnifies. The by-products of glycation
accumulate in the body and skin constantly appears
dull and aged.'

Dull and aged, versus the red and teenaged complexion my
detox had given me. It was a tough choice. But I packed my
concealer, picked up my bag and headed off to work, hoping
this would only be temporary.

Day three, like the day before, passed in a haze. I didn't feel
hungry – I'd brought oatcakes and a sliced avocado to snack
on, plus a handful of almonds to eat at around 4 p.m. when
I know I always have the urge to graze. Lunch was another
salad, this time with turkey, spinach, beetroot and other bits
and pieces, topped off with a drizzling of plain olive oil. The
food itself didn't feel at all like a sacrifice, but I very much
missed my fizzy pop and smoothies. By the time 7.30 p.m.

rolled around I was ready for bed. My head was pounding and I felt as if someone had filled my head with helium. I took another taxi home (this getting healthy thing was expensive) and, after I'd eaten a spinach frittata, taken my make-up off and daubed my copious spots with giant blobs of Sudocrem (the benefits of being single, again) I climbed straight to bed. But yet again I couldn't sleep.

This was getting ridiculous.

It must have been about three hours later at around midnight that I finally drifted off, only to be plagued by strange abstract dreams including one involving a massive lobster. I woke up at 5 a.m., clammy and exhausted, and rather pathetically, I started to cry.

There are few things guaranteed to make you feel more lonely than waking up, on your own, in the middle of the night while everyone else – possibly in the whole universe (or so it feels) – is asleep, to angst over a huge life-change you're making. I kept asking myself what I was trying to achieve through all of this. Thinness? Absurd levels of health? Because there was no such thing as eternal life and I've always been determined to strike a balance between enjoyment and virtue. Several friends had already tutted and muttered the immortal words 'life's too short' when I told them why I wasn't indulging in something or another over the past few days. I started to wonder if it was all worth the effort.

Part of my malaise was a touch of the detox-related blues,

I knew that. My body was in the midst of an huge chemical, behavioural and physical transformation, and feeling a little unsettled and odd was natural. But there was also a large part of me that wasn't really sure why I was putting myself through this. While I was on the large side of normal, I wasn't someone who felt massively aggrieved by their size. I was happy with my life and my lifestyle, so why was I upsetting the apple cart, isolating myself and changing my entire social life? Regardless of how slim I became, how would I ever meet another boyfriend if I never went out for drinks or to dinner? And more to the point, how long would these horrendous feelings of illness last?

I felt so down in the dumps and sick, I decided to take the day off work, which was practically unheard of. Looking back now, I know day four was my lowest point. Subsequent research has also taught me that these feelings are an important and intrinsic part of human psychology when it comes to giving something up. Overblown dramatic feelings of doubt like these are your brain's way of making sure you really want to make the change you are about to make – a subject I will explore further in Chapter Eight.

Whether it was the withdrawal, the lack of sleep or a combination of all those things, I felt incredibly faint. I had an upset stomach and took to the sofa for the whole day to watch Wimbledon, but was unable to concentrate on anything. In the afternoon I took a stroll to the nearby shops and accidentally stepped out in front of a car on the way there *and* the way back. I stared at a workman drinking a can of Coke and was so incredibly jealous of the treacly, bubbly joyousness of drinking it I almost asked for a sip.

At a loss, I got home and went on the internet for support. Many others who'd given up sugar advised drinking copious amounts of water to help your body eliminate the toxins. Although I already drank a litre and a half each day, many said to aim for two and a half litres daily during your detox, minimum. Hurrah! This was something I could do. Others suggested light exercise like a walk around the park. I also decided to make something nice for dinner and to do an online shop to fill my cupboards with hearty healthy foods where there were currently just depressingly empty shelves.

For me, a healthy diet isn't measured by what you don't eat but by what you do. There's no point cutting back on your sugars to cover things in honey and the like. Or, instead of eating full-sugar versions of things, going for an artificially sweetened alternative. That's not going to improve your health much.

No, nutritious food is what will improve your health, so I began filling my virtual trolley with nuts. Lots of nuts was what I needed. And cinnamon, seeds, organic whole yoghurt, rice milk, herbal teas, brown rice, spelt pasta, eggs, hummus, pulses, plenty of organic oak-smoked salmon, mackerel and grains.

I decided that when I was cooking for myself, I'd try to eat only organic dairy produce, meat and fish. While it's much more expensive, I'd reasoned that I'd rather eat meat less often, but eat better, healthier, happier meat that's not been pumped full of antibiotics. Dark green vegetables, fizzy water, good-quality olive oils for salads and almond nut butter went into the trolley. Avocados too. Coconut oil to cook with and the desiccated stuff to add to my new favourite recipe: protein pancakes (see Chapter Six, page 185). Sweet potatoes. Spaghetti made from spelt for dietary emergencies when I need something quick and filling. And I realised I needed to expand my spice rack, bearing in mind that most of my flavours would now be coming from here after sauces had been eliminated. I was buoyed by the fact that there was a lot I could eat, lots of really good stuff, but four things struck me:

◆ This new healthy Nicole was going to be expensive to run.

◆ I had to learn to become a better cook, sharpish.

◆ Most recipes you make from scratch don't contain sugar anyhow.

◆ Why hadn't someone told me that quinoa was pronounced keen-wah before I trudged into the health food shop and made a prat out of myself?

That night I had a bath with some Aromatherapy Associates Deep Relax oil (nope, not Ryan Gosling) and packed myself off to bed at about 10 p.m. It was a Friday night, so another very rock and roll evening.

Again, I slept fitfully and had to get up twice to go to the loo (damn that water drinking advice), but if I wasn't mistaken, the next day my headache had started to abate. Still, I lay on the sofa most of the day, but managed to get the energy up to go to the cinema with my friend Katy in the afternoon. Big mistake. The smell of popcorn was almost overwhelmingly good. I drooled my way through *Prometheus* while a man next to me ate a miniature pot of toffee-flavoured ice cream. I stomped home in a real grump before making a cinnamon and cardamom tea that I hoped would help soothe away my cravings.

If that little outing taught me anything it's that abstinence is much harder in the face of temptation. Until I was feeling mentally stronger, I resolved not to put myself in the position of being around things that I missed. There are few things less fun than sitting in a cinema salivating into someone else's popcorn. Plus, at this early stage I couldn't trust myself not to crack were someone to encourage me to have, say a KitKat or a large glass of Sancerre. Or a KitKat and a glass of Sancerre.

By the time Sunday came around, my headache had evaporated. I woke up once in the night but, mindful not to let feelings of anger and worry overtake me, went straight back to sleep. I attended a gentle yoga class at the gym and, after my big supermarket order had come and I'd replenished my cupboards, I made an Asian beef salad with lots of beansprouts and shredded vegetables.

Monday and, with only a minor headache behind the eyes, a box of a dozen cupcakes from the legendary cake-maker The Hummingbird Bakery, arrived at work addressed to me. For some perverse reason, press officers often send giant boxes of cakes, biscuits, chocolates or doughnuts to women who work in the fashion, health and beauty departments of magazines and newspapers. They seem to feel that some of the most weight-obsessed women on the planet will appreciate these 'little treats', which arrive on a daily basis from somewhere or another. Indeed, I liked to call these types of gifts a box of 'diet mockers' (while often eating the icing off the top of one). Yet on this day I placed them on an empty desk as far away from my seat as possible. I knew there was nothing to fear with this strategy. If you're not quick as a flash, the 30-or-so women I worked with would see to it that there was no temptation left to succumb to.

While supportive, some work colleagues had been somewhat mystified about my new regime (I was careful not to use the word 'diet' as I saw what I was doing as a holistic change for my health rather than just my waistline). 'Just have half with me' some would plead as they went down to the canteen to get a chocolate bar at 4 p.m. I realised that my order of a peppermint tea when others were indulging was probably rather hard to stomach. When one person begins abstaining from the communal sweet round, it makes you feel as if you are being judged.

Unfortunately though, I am a people pleaser. Left to my own devices my willpower will rarely falter; put me in a room with people exuding a sense of disappointment that I'm not doing something or other, and I'll almost certainly buckle, just to keep the peace.

Worried I would crack, I explained to the team that they needed to help me stay on the straight and narrow and my ever-supportive colleague Olivia immediately went out and bought a bag of nuts for us to share on the desk. I could have cried with joy.

But there's definitely a competitive element towards food in all-female offices too – and it's something that's not specific to the women of the media. Both my mum and sister work for the NHS and when I asked if 'who was eating what and when' was debated around their photocopier too, they looked at me as if I were an imbecile. 'Of course it is,' they said. 'Everyone has an office feeder. Have you ever tried refusing a piece of their homemade cake?' asked my sister Natalie. 'That's pressure.'

Tuesday, one week in, I started to feel better. I'd got the snacking thing down pat; chopping up vegetables before work and taking them in with a small pot of hummus. It was an effort, but it was worth it and my friend Kate also got in on the act, bringing in her own veggie dippers and pots of hummus, which made it almost fun. I realised it was vitally important I always had a little pack of trusty oatcakes in my bag in case hunger should urgently and unexpectedly strike. Avocados became ridiculously important to me as an afternoon snack, and my morning coffee (bought, without fail, from a great little independent shop on my way into work each morning) was the treat that would see me through until lunchtime.

The deep and regular sleep that had been my default setting until the last few years had returned, which suddenly made everything seem bearable. I somehow found the energy to slowly cycle my Pashley bicycle home from work, where it had been languishing in the basement car park for nearly a week, although it did take me 10 minutes longer than usual.

And from there the days began passing relatively painlessly. I summoned up the courage to buy a paper from Nina's corner shop at the end of my road, which I'd been avoiding it as it meant confronting row upon row of chocolate bars and a divine little area of penny sweets. The worst of my spots had begun to disappear and, on Friday, a colleague commented that the whites of my eyes looked brighter. It's a pretty strange compliment, granted (were they yellow before?) and it wasn't something I'd noticed myself, but I was desperate for any kind of sign that this regime was working. The next week too, another guy in the office said my eyes looked twinkly. Unless this was some bizarre office prank, it became obvious that whatever changes were going on inside my body, they were obviously affecting my peepers first.

I'd read in various books and on some websites that other people who had quit sugar had started to feel well after three days, then amazing and bursting with energy after about five. I asked Ian why he thought it could have taken me so much longer to start even feeling okay, let alone 'amazing':

'Most people feel quite ill for about three days,' he said. 'The fact that you felt ill longer could be because you were perhaps slightly insulin resistant.'

This was interesting. In 2013, I had found out that – like one in five women in the UK – I have polycystic ovarian syndrome (PCOS). In case you're unfamiliar, PCOS sufferers simply have more follicles – or cysts – on their ovaries. Like me, half of the women with PCOS have no symptoms and may never realise they have the condition unless they have an ultrasound scan, but there are links between it and so-called insulin resistance. We've already learnt earlier in this chapter that insulin is a hormone produced by the pancreas to deal with high amounts of glucose (sugar) in the blood. It essentially allows glucose into the cells to be used as energy. If you have a degree of insulin resistance (it's measured on a sliding scale) your body will not react quickly to insulin and the pancreas will keep making more of the hormone to try and keep blood sugar regulated. Eventually, the body's cells stop responding to insulin and glucose builds up in the blood, leading to diabetes.

Some evidence points to women with PCOS having a higher risk of type 2 diabetes in later life. While I didn't have any testing done at the time so it would be impossible to now tell if I had a degree of insulin resistance when I was eating a high sugar diet, perhaps it would be useful for you to know the symptoms, to see if you could benefit from a few blood tests. Here goes:

Insulin resistance indicators

Brain fogginess – check

High blood sugar – unsure as I wasn't tested at the time

Intestinal bloating – sorry, not very glamorous but, check

Sleepiness, especially after meals – not so much after meals, but I did generally need a lot of sleep

Weight gain, fat storage, difficulty losing weight – check, check, check

Increased levels of blood triglycerides (fats in the blood) – unknown

Increased blood pressure – yes, my blood pressure had always been on the high side of normal

High cholesterol – no

Increased levels of pro-inflammatory cytokines in the blood (the proteins which cause cellular inflammation) – unknown

Depression – while I have periods of feeling down, I wouldn't call it depression, so no

Darker patches of skin under the armpits, on the neck or on the body's skin folds – no

Increased hunger – yes definitely

In the coming days, I started to notice other changes too. Bizarrely, my sense of smell had gone crazy. While I've never been a fan of Red Bull, a super-sweet waft coming from the open can of the guy next to me on the Tube made me feel ill. I could smell chocolate muffins cooking in the bakery part of the supermarket from the entrance to the store (they smelled alarmingly great too). Diet Coke smelled strangely metallic… it was as if the scents of things had become magnified.

Almost two weeks in was when I first received a compliment about my skin. At a work breakfast meeting, a contact said I looked 'glowing'. My clothes had become looser – something that had been noticed by several women in my office – and my stomach flatter, which was probably down to the fact that my formerly sluggish digestion had ramped up not just one but several gears. I suppose upping your veg intake will do that to a girl.

Truth be told, my bad moods had also been because I'd been secretly seething for the past few weeks that I couldn't eat what I wanted. While some women can snack on chocolate after having a burger for lunch and still stay a size 10, that just wasn't me. It wasn't ever going to be me and I had to accept it. I'd been feeling hard done-by, and while that feeling had not gone away, around week three, I started to feel less moody. Urban legend has it that it takes 21 days to break an old habit or make a new one and for me, this certainly seemed to be accurate. Don't get me wrong, I was still furious about the fact that I was unable to eat chocolate like many friends who seemed to be able to trough it down and not put on a pound; but I felt generally less stressed. I'm part Irish and have definitely inherited my dad's fiery temper, but by week three, I started to feel as if I were able to take things more in my stride. While a month before, a writer missing a deadline or never answering their phone was liable to send me into a furious rant, it now felt less important, or at least not important enough to get myself worked up about.

The easiest way to put it is this: whereas I'd previously felt as if I'd been on a mood rollercoaster, I suddenly felt as if I'd got off the ride. My energy levels had stabilised too – no more mid-morning and teatime slumps when I felt I 'needed' to have a biscuit or three. I felt liberated. At the time, I couldn't really explain why, it was just something I noticed.

I decided to look into the possibility of a link between stress and sugar. As many of us can attest, there's nothing like a difficult time to send us straight to the tuck box. The latest stats show that over the last 50 years – as lives in the Western world have become increasingly stressful – our consumption of processed sugar has tripled. According to the International Cocoa Foundation, Britons each consume a staggering 24 lb of chocolate alone every year – and that's before you factor in any other sweet treats or any sugars hidden in processed foods.

However, far from the stress buster many of us credit them with being, research suggests that sugary treats actually cause us to become *more* panicked and wired rather than less, which could explain my change in mood since giving them up.

Scientists at the charity Food for the Brain (a group of doctors, scientists, nutritionists, psychiatrists and psychologists who aim to promote the link between food and mental health) believe there is a relationship between behavioural changes and the levels of sugar in our blood.

'There is a direct link between mood and blood sugar balance,' Deborah Colson, a nutritional therapist for the charity told me when I spoke to her. 'Our experience is that poor blood sugar balance is often the single biggest factor in people suffering mood swings, depression, anxiety and what I call "emotionality" – which is someone who appears to be fine one minute, then in floods of tears the next. Having big blood sugar swings lessens people's ability to cope with stress.

'There are of course lots of factors in modern life that contribute to stress and low moods (the breakdown of family structures is one example) but bad diet is a big factor. Nutrient-rich foods are essential for good mental health – B vitamins, zinc, magnesium,

chromium, essential fatty acids – and people who eat
diets high in sugar just won't be giving their bodies
the right coping mechanisms.'

I've already mentioned that my job was incredibly stressful.
Long hours are not only hard to handle when you're in the
office, but also mean that when you aren't, you rush around
trying to fit in all the things you should have done when you
were at work – cleaning the house, seeing friends, picking
up your dry cleaning, going to the shops… It dawned on me
that I was probably existing on adrenaline and cortisol – the
so-called 'fight or flight' hormones – that your body releases
naturally when you're under pressure. As well as causing
you to lay down fat around your waist and tummy, excessive
adrenaline and cortisol production makes the body crave
sugar – and excess sugar then makes you feel stressed.

Learning this made it easier to see sugar for what it was: a
wolf in sheep's clothing. I knew then that my sugar-free trial,
as I'd been billing it to make it less scary, had to be more than
that. Given what I now knew, I didn't think I would ever be
able to go back to my old ways.

Yet there were wobbles. Just under two weeks in, my dad and
I went to the women's semi-finals at Wimbledon. The matches
started at lunchtime and when we met at the entrance of the
All-England Club, it became apparent fairly rapidly that there
was basically nothing I could eat. Strawberries and cream?

Nope. Champagne? Er, no thanks. I knew I should have let Mum make us a picnic, as she had been insisting. Instead, I ended up getting a posh hot-dog for about a tenner, eating the sausage and leaving the bun. It was hardly the most nutritious lunch. Dad thought I'd lost the plot.

Likewise, the weekend just before my three-week anniversary I decided to drive to Henley to see Aspen, an old friend and housemate from university who now lived out in the countryside with her boyfriend, baby daughter and their dog. I set off, got stuck in a whopping traffic jam and then nearly ran out of petrol. At the services, already an hour and a half late for lunch, I was famished and felt strange. I wanted a snack. But could I find anything? Could I hell. The drinks fridge didn't even have any plain water left, only Volvic Touch of Fruit Lemon and Lime flavoured water, which, with 27 g of sugar in a 500 ml bottle (the equivalent of 7 teaspoons, or three Krispy Kreme doughnuts) isn't something I fancied drinking after I'd done so well. I cursed myself for not having any oatcakes and instead bought some dry-roasted peanuts and a can of Diet Coke. One sip and I threw the drink away. How I ever managed to get through a couple of cans of this stuff a day is beyond me. It tasted so strange, a combination of overly sweet and metallic. Of course, I inhaled all the peanuts before I'd got back onto the motorway. They were dreamy.

But back to the new me, emerging like a big butterfly from a spotty chrysalis. Obvious changes had begun to take place. My nails seemed to be growing faster and stronger. My skin was already so much better. Without make-up on I had rosy cheeks again, rather than the sallow grey blotchy complexion I'd become accustomed to. My taste buds had gone into overdrive. Things that didn't used to taste sweet – milk, almonds – took on a whole new flavour for me. While the life-altering changes – a revamped immune system, a complete transformation of my menstrual cycle – would happen gradually, over the coming weeks and months (more on this later in the book), my clothes felt looser, indeed some friends commented that I looked as if I had been 'vacuum packed'… all the better as I was going on holiday to Spain in four weeks' time. This would be the biggest test yet.

Chapter Three

FAMILY TIES

The realisation that I wouldn't be going back to the old me was both liberating and scary because, to paraphrase John Candy in *Trains, Planes and Automobiles* (a seminal film from my childhood), 'I liked me'.

I was the girl with six bottles of champagne in her fridge, 10 beers, 20 bottles of expensive nail polishes of varying shades (here's a little tip: keeping nail polish in the fridge helps slow down any colour fading, and means it paints on more smoothly) and little else aside from milk, perhaps some eggs, parmesan and spinach. Those were the ingredients needed for a good night in, and I was fine with that. Most of my friends were the same – women, in our early thirties, all of whom had done well in our careers, mostly lived on our own and did what we liked, when we liked, with whom we liked.

But now my life needed planning. I had to organise what I would eat for breakfast, lunch and dinner in advance to ensure I had the ingredients in the house. Kicking the habit wasn't only going to involve a complete change of eating habits, but also a lifestyle overhaul.

The new me had a fridge full of jars of tahini (a sesame seed paste used to make dressings) and bottles of cider apple vinegar, salad crispers full of cucumbers, beetroots, peppers, celery, kale and anything else hearty I could get my hands on. Gone was the ever-present large bar of dark Montezuma's chocolate that was replenished every time it got down to the final few squares. There were almond and hemp seed butters where the beers used to be. Plain organic oatcakes instead of dark chocolate digestives. The freezer was empty apart from ice trays, peas and some organic chicken breasts I'd put in there before they went off. My bank balance was groaning under the strain of all the fresh produce I was loading up on.

A month in, I was still going strong, but I hated the idea of any type of food being 'naughty' or somehow 'not allowed'. People who express faux horror at eating half a cupcake have always made me want to stab myself in the eye so I was determined not to become one of them. If you want it, eat it. Don't make a big deal about it and don't lament it after it's passed your lips.

But then here was I, being the most faddy restrictive eater I'd ever known and actually rather liking it. From day one, I'd made a rule not to tell people about my regime unless they noticed or asked. I couldn't be bothered to explain the whys and the wherefores to business contacts or people I was casually meeting for breakfast or lunch. It always initiates a monologue from me which leaves me feeling like I have monopolised the conversation – which I often have. Besides, I've always felt uncomfortable about admitting to being on 'a diet'. Perhaps it's because I feel it shows that you're unhappy with yourself in some way, that you want to change yourself. Although I wanted to slim down and get healthy, I didn't want people to think I was 'unhappy' with myself.

Remarkably, however, very few people actually noticed that I was restricting my sugar intake when I was out with them for dinner. It wasn't immediately apparent when I was ordering. Things that are sweet are actually quite easy to identify and avoid. And that's the great thing about going low sugar, choose your restaurant wisely and you can eat just about anything from any menu (not desserts though – kiss those goodbye). My favourites – such as fish or smoked salmon – followed by steak and a salad is just fine. Likewise, stir-fries with brown (if possible) rice. Roast dinners are great, stews, barbecues, salads (be careful with the dressing). It's easy to see why strangers didn't notice I was following any kind of eating plan at all.

But, I needed to tell my parents about giving up sugar. While I'd got away with it at Wimbledon with my dad, there was no way abstinence would escape the eagle eyes of my mum. I'd resisted up until this point as I didn't think she would understand. My mum is amazing, caring, literally the best mum anyone could ask for, but sometimes it feels as if

'Living Up In London' makes her worry that I'll fall foul of some sort of strange food cult. Even before I gave up sugar, she often checked in with what I'm eating, exclaiming that I 'need to eat more than just that' despite my being a more than healthy size. Or she asks 'but where is your fibre coming from?' when I tell her what I had for lunch. Indeed, when my parents come to visit, Mum often brings a pint of milk or some tea bags with her from home. Or she'll bring a spaghetti bolognaise sauce that she's made and frozen, transporting it on the train wrapped in a food bag and five plastic carrier bags so that the other passengers don't smell it as it defrosts. If I happen to mention I've tried something new that I like – coconut-flavoured yoghurts were one thing – mum would bring up a pack of four each time she visits. I tell her we do have food in London, and I can make my own spaghetti bolognaise, yet she persists. Bless her, it's as if Sussex and its hearty fayre is a world away, rather than just 50 miles down the M23.

But while Mum has always been militant about draining off the fat from anything she's cooking and not adding salt to foods – her catchphrase being: 'it already has all the salt it needs in it naturally' – there seemed to be no such restrictions on sugar. Adding it to drinks was not allowed, but consuming it in things seemed to go unnoticed.

While it's not a regular occurrence, my family can inhale a box of Maltesers in one sitting. Like many kids who grew up in the eighties, there was never really an issue with drinking pints of sugary squash. Biscuits were readily available, as were fizzy drinks at the weekend. Unsurprisingly, both Natalie and I had quite a lot of fillings as children.

Sweets were definitely used to mark milestones. At Christmas, the Mowbrays will get through two tins of Roses (Mum buys boxes to replenish the tin when it gets empty). When my sister and I were growing up, Dad played rugby on a Saturday afternoon, so Mum, Nanny, Natalie and I would go 'down town' where we had this ritual: when all the shopping and chores had been done, Nanny would buy each of us a bar of clotted cream fudge from Thorntons which we'd eat on the way home. Mmmmmm, fudge.

So, three weeks in, during one of my nightly phone calls home, I dropped the no-sugar bombshell:

'I've given up eating sugar, Mum,' I said.

'But you don't eat any sugar,' came her reply.

'Well, I do,' said I. 'It's in cereals and fruit and sauces. Bread and drinks – alcohol – and ice cream and pretty much all the things I like, so I'm cutting it out.'

Silence.

'And fruit juice and smoothies. It's in so many things, it's terrifying,' I continued.

'Riiiight,' Mum replied. 'Well, you have to eat fruit and cereals. And fruit juices and smoothies. Is this one of those silly low-carb things? Because brown bread is good for you.

Fruit and juices are good for you, there's nothing wrong with those. You're basically saying there's nothing you can eat, which is just silly. You won't get enough vitamins and you'll feel unwell. Everything in moderation is fine. Besides, you do have to live and enjoy your life, not just exist.'

It was at this point I decided to agree and leave the conversation there. It was probably something best introduced gradually and in person, when she could see I was in no danger of either wasting away or dying of scurvy any time soon. Not long after our chat ended, my metaphorical ears started burning. Right now, the information – 'Nicole's gone on a silly fad diet' – would be being passed on to my dad and sister (now married and living two streets away with her first daughter, Millie) – 'she's not even eating *bread*'.

Mum's reaction hadn't shocked me. The detox had taught me many things, but the most powerful was that you don't need to eat chocolate every day or add sugar to your tea or syrup to your coffee to be sugar dependent. I had been a secret sweet fiend, and it was probable that my whole family were too – not to the same extent as they didn't drink juices by the gallon or slurp Diet Cokes throughout the day.

Although I spared them the lecture, I decided to take a look into whether having a sweet tooth has been found to be genetic. I mean, do you inherit your tastes or are they learnt? There has actually been quite a lot of research on this very subject and all the evidence points towards the fact that having a sweet tooth is genetic. Research by scientists at the University of Toronto has identified that some people have a variation in a gene called 'Glucose Transporter Type Two' (abbreviated to GLUT2) and those people consistently consume more sugar than people without the variation.

It wasn't hard to see where I'd got mine. Both my nanny and grandma (both now deceased) had incredibly sweet teeth. Perhaps it was because both of them lived through the war and rationing, but Nan took four spoons of sugar in her tea and coffee until the late 1960s, and Grandma was the same. Mum's dad (who died when she was 15) also, apparently, took heaps in his drinks. Dad's father died when my dad was seven.

> 'When rationing ended and sugar was freely available again, people apparently went crazy for it,' Dad told me. 'Grandma said that as soon as it was available again, she satisfied a seven-year craving for pineapple in syrup by buying two large tins and eating both straight out of the tin with a spoon. She was violently ill and never touched pineapple again that I can recall.'

Not that that put her off sugar in all forms. Indeed, Grandma also used to eat bread and butter with sugar on it for breakfast and her beloved bread, butter and suet raisin roly-poly puddings were topped with both golden syrup and sugar. Unsurprisingly, she also had a full set of upper and lower dentures.

My dad also developed a sweet tooth at an early age. Being the only boy after five girls and the youngest, he admits he was 'heartily spoilt', getting virtually unlimited sweets and the like from his older siblings and his many aunts and uncles (Dad's mum, my grandma, was Irish Catholic and the youngest of 13 children). His mid-morning snack was a bar of Five Boys chocolate, which he used to eat in the back garden with his dog Sally.

> 'Many kids at that time were lacking in basic nutrition and mums were encouraged to stuff supplements into them at any opportunity,' Dad says. 'I fell in love with something called "Cod Liver Oil and Malt", a thick glutinous substance which must have tasted foul in its raw state, so I suspect it was lavishly dosed with sugar to make it palatable. It lived in the top of the larder in a large brown jar with a screw-on, brass-coloured lid. I took 2 tablespoons at night – the second being almost impossible to get off the spoon – then straight to bed with no thoughts of tooth brushing. This was back in the good old 1950s. I also distinctly recall eating Lyle's Golden Syrup straight out of the green and gold tin with a tablespoon.'

Dewsbury Library

Tel: (01484) 414 868
Email: Dewsbury.lic@kirklees.gov.uk

Customer ID: *****7121

Items that you have borrowed

Title: Breaking up with sugar : a plan to divorce
the diets, drop the pounds and live your
best life
ID: 800758100
Due: 09 November 2022

Title: Men's health : all you need to know in
one concise manual
ID: 800739886
Due: 09 November 2022

Title: Sweet nothing : why I gave up sugar and
how you can too
ID: 800467953
Due: 09 November 2022

Total items: 3
Checked out: 3
Overdue: 0
Hold requests: 0
Ready for collection: 0
19/10/2022 11:22

Thank you for using the bibliotheca SelfCheck
System.
We hope to see you soon.

www.kirklees.gov.uk/community/libraries

Mum – who used to have banana and sugar sandwiches as a regular sugar fix – says she gave up adding sugar to drinks in the late 1960s after both she and her mum suffered from stomach aches and, for some reason, decided sugar was the cause. By the time my parents met in 1971, Dad says Mum was 'diluting the Fanta and Coca-Cola she was drinking with liberal amounts of Bacardi'.

But apparently, when I was born, followed by my sister Natalie two years later, the house was virtually a sugar-free zone. Indeed, Dad used to call sugar 'white poison'. No one added sugar to drinks or food, but somewhere along the line – whether it was when the population began eating processed food, or when scoffing junk food became the norm – we all began to lose track of exactly how much of the white stuff we were eating, hence Mum's idea that I didn't really eat any sugar simply because I didn't add it to food or drinks.

'Most processed food has sugar added to it, sometimes from several sources,' Ian Marber told me. 'If you look at the ingredients list on a packet, the biggest is meant to be added first. Sometimes you'll find that the list could read "water, sugar," then something else, making sugar the second biggest ingredient...

'Sugars give an interest to a product that would be entirely bland otherwise. It's as if our tastes have become numbed to everything. It's not enough to just have something that is slightly sweet, it needs to be overwhelmingly sweet.

'When I tell clients not to have sushi but instead have sashimi and a side of brown rice, they don't understand the difference. I tell them that to make the rice sticky, it has to have sugar added to it.

'Other surprising places that you'll find sugar include in things like high-fibre bread. Indeed, things that are perceived as healthy often contain quite a lot of sugar – granola is an obvious one, Rachel's Organic Low Fat Vanilla Yogurt contains more sugar than it does vanilla... Things that sound very healthy are sometimes the worst culprits. You probably wouldn't give your child Frosties because you know that they're full of sugar. But perhaps you would give them good-quality muesli like Dorset Cereals. Yet many varieties of this are also incredibly high in sugar. We know that a can of Coke contains a hefty dose of sugar – 35 g – and a Mars Bar has 30 g. That's not shocking.

'But perhaps you'd think that a Rachel's Organic Fat-Free Blueberry Yogurt would be nothing but good for you? After all, there are four implied health claims in the Rachel's packaging – "organic", "fat-free", "blueberry" and "yogurt". It's probable that many parents would rather their child had that than, say, a Müller Crunch Strawberry Shortcake Yogurt, which contains 17.5 g of sugar per 100 g (which is considered a medium amount of sugar, by the way).

'You may be surprised then to learn then, that the Rachel's Organic Fat-Free Blueberry Yogurt contains 13.9 g of sugar per 100 g – not much less than the Müller product. At least the Strawberry Shortcake Yogurt is what it says it is, and doesn't pretend to be healthy. Many of us shop on autopilot, but we need to look at the words on the food labels that we are putting in our cupboards.'

Ian is right, may of us do shop on autopilot, habitually picking up the same items that we think are good for us without any more examination. I know I did and would frequently eat the same things day after day – granola for breakfast, sushi for lunch, snacking on grapes and dried fruit, ordering the same smoothie, making the same stir-fries or risottos for dinner. But while being aware of what we're eating is one thing, having the strength not to eat what you desire is another.

I'd never had that drive to quit sugar before, but now I did. I was really spurred on by the rapid weight loss I was experiencing – over half a stone in the first month without really feeling hungry or deprived.

This was important, because, Lord knows, I have never been good with hunger. Nine years ago, my friend Nell and I went to the exclusive Chiva Som health retreat in Thailand; I was writing about it for the newspaper we were both working for at the time. It was a gruelling 12-hour flight that arrived into Bangkok early in the morning the following day. We'd got unexpectedly upgraded and had a couple of glasses of wine on the flight – nothing too major, but that, combined with no sleep, meant I felt horrible as we waited for our luggage in the refrigerated arrivals hall. Being jostled out into the hideous sweatbox that was Bangkok in the morning rush hour did not help.

Chiva Som is near to the coastal resort of Hua Hin, a town patronised by the Thai royal family who have a summer home there. It's about a three-hour drive from the capital. A beautiful heavenly place, right on the beach but lush, green and tropical. Little wonder that celebrities and captains of industry return, year after year to hunker down for a week and get their body and minds back on track. We arrived, were handed cool lemongrass towels and a delicious iced tea before being escorted to our luxurious room. I was famished, we both were, and after a helper had shown us everything under the sun: 'this is how to open the wardrobe [opens wardrobe normally]… this is how to shut the wardrobe [again, shuts it normally]… and here's how you open the patio door' [yep, a sliding door, we get it], I hurried him out and made for the minibar.

The only thing inside it was a batch of homemade raw carob brownies. Basically what I – at the time – considered fake chocolate brownies. And water. There was plenty of water. While today I'd view raw carob brownies as a special occasion snack, back in 2005, I couldn't believe the worthiness of it. While I didn't care about the lack of booze, there was no soda pop, no pricey Pringles or expensive tiny jars of nuts. The obligatory foreign KitKat was absent, as were the £8 packet of peanut M&Ms you'd stuff down at 5 a.m. when your brain thinks it's midnight and your stomach thinks it's midday. We ate the welcome brownies. They were not replenished.

I felt panicked. But, we were on a luxury health retreat; they weren't about to let us faint from hunger. And indeed they did not. We went to the restaurant, ate lots of fresh healthy food, and spent the rest of the day dozing, dribbling and jolting ourselves awake on the sunbeds.

Then, the detox programme began. It was what I had gone there to write about so I shouldn't have been surprised, but overnight we were required to do a full fast (no food or water) so the resort's doctors could test our blood and saliva to determine which programme to put us on. The next morning when the tests came around, Nell was so parched she couldn't summon up enough spit (it couldn't have bubbles, those were the rules) to even fill the little testing pot. I felt bleak. My programme involved just drinking broth with some sort-of coriander leaves floating in it twice a day and a light meal in the evening. Occasional chunks of papaya (which I thought tasted like cheese) were allowed. There was unlimited water and herbal tea but little else. Consequently, I was in the foulest of moods all day and went to bed at about 6 p.m. The next day I was grumpy and tearful and I wanted to go home. Plus, we were to begin a programme of daily colonic irrigations. But happily, I knew something they didn't. That morning while unpacking, I'd found a jumbo-sized bag of Fox's Glacier Fruits – again, mad for sweets even then – that I'd bought for the plane, at the bottom of my cabin bag. Nell was strong, but I duly proceeded to eat them throughout the next three days, putting the wrappers back into a pocket of my suitcase so I wouldn't get rumbled – not that anyone would have, after all I was only cheating myself. One day we took a tuk-tuk into town and bought some Dorito-type crisps from a Tesco store we found (I know, they have Tesco over there!), eating them all before we got back to the hotel. When we left, lighter and brighter after five days of not having ingested anything of significant calorific value, we went to Bangkok for a few days and straight to a McDonald's. Yes, Chiva Som was gorgeous, the treatments were amazing and we were thinner with flat tummies and glowing skin, but because food is a key part of my enjoyment of life, all I could remember was spending four or five days feeling famished.

There was no way I would ever be able to stick to a diet that left me feeling hungry for lots of the time. But giving up sugar hadn't. I'd found that I could still eat plenty of food, just food that was completely different.

I'll go into what I ate in more detail later in the book, but here's a sample day.

Wake up: a pint of water

Breakfast: a bowl of organic plain yoghurt, sprinkled with ground nuts, a few oats, some linseeds and a sprinkling of cinnamon

Lunch: a big turkey salad with tomatoes, spinach and lots of leaves, an egg, pine nuts, dressed with olive oil

Afternoon snack: some avocado on oatcakes

Dinner: a steak salad and plain yoghurt for pudding

Six weeks in and as I was feeling strong, I decided to go out to a friend's leaving drinks party. It was billed as a sedate affair, at a pub in central London. 'Pop along after work,' the email said, and so I did. By the time I arrived, it was 7.45 and the assembled crowd were in fine fettle; or what some may term 'loud'. I immediately knew this was a bad idea. No one would understand why I wasn't drinking and it would all be horribly awkward, but just as I was debating whether to leave before I got spotted, I got spotted.

'Coley!' came the shout, 'Get over here! Wow, you look amazing. What have you been doing?' asked my friend Jen, who was now in the process of summoning over other mutual friends so they could examine the new slimline me. I wasn't eating sugar, I explained as someone handed me an empty wine glass and proceeded to fill it up with doubtless bad house white from a bottle standing in one of the many ice buckets dotted around a large table.

'Oooh, er no thanks,' I said, handing back the glass. 'I'm alright for wine, I'm not really drinking tonight,' I explained, to looks of puzzlement. 'No, I'm not pregnant,' I said, in answer to the many quizzical remarks, 'it's just, alcohol – especially beer and white wine – is mostly sugar so I'm avoiding it at the moment.'

Talk about a buzz-killer. I could see their eyes glaze over. I was stood in a pub, saying that drinking was bad for you. So, I went to the bar and got myself a single vodka with fresh lime and soda water. It was my first alcoholic drink in about six weeks and I took a sip. The familiar, slightly antiseptic taste of the spirit hit my tongue immediately, followed by a rush of tartness from the lime. Vodka, lime and soda isn't only incredibly low in calories and sugar, it's also not moreish – perhaps because it's not particularly nice. Two sips in, I ditched the straw as I'd started to feel slightly lightheaded and strange. As I nursed my drink, I noticed the group getting louder and louder and their drunken conversations becoming progressively harder to follow. A third sip and I decided to sneak off home. So, like all good journalists, I made my excuses and left, abandoning my half-drunk drink and my half-cut friends.

I spent the journey home pondering how I could make going out palatable again when I'm not drinking to get drunk. Perhaps I'd have to drive to events, or maybe arrive early and leave early, before everyone gets a bit obnoxious.

Yet, seeing friends I hadn't seen for months and being on the receiving end of their compliments had spurred me on. Everyone without fail said I looked healthy. Many commented that my skin looked good, all commented on the weight that I had lost. This, like nothing else, had brought it home to me that eating sugar just didn't agree with me. After recounting my family's love of the white stuff it's not hard to see where I got my taste for sugar from, but the rest of the family were slender. I was not.

Even at school, despite copious amounts of exercise – competitive swimming training at a club twice a week, netball for the school twice weekly, doing an evening paper round on my bike and taking a GCSE in PE (I know, and yes you can get a qualification in PE), I was still a tubby teen. I'd fallen into bad habits – eating McDonald's with friends in town on Saturday, followed by copious amounts of pick-n-mix and strawberry bootlaces from Woolworths. I became an expert pesterer, harangued Mum for Frosties for breakfast and bags of Iced Gems to put in my packed lunch. I would sneak packets of Party Rings biscuits – the ones covered in multi-coloured icing – into the trolley at Sainsbury's and promptly commandeer them when we got home, taking them upstairs and inhaling the whole lot in one sitting. It can't have been easy having such a piglet for a daughter and as I was then at high school, 'working' (doing a paper round) and earning my own pocket money – all of which was spent on sweets and clothes – the matter was slipping out of their control.

Yet my sister was the exact opposite. Natalie was famed in our family for doing anything to get out of eating meals, including one famous incident on holiday in America whereby she 'dropped' a burger under the table and pretended she had eaten it. She was only rumbled when Dad – who'd slipped his sandals off – promptly squidged his foot into a lukewarm beef patty covered in ketchup. It didn't go down well.

Natalie and I were both raised in very similar ways, yet we had polar opposite tastes and attitudes to food. So, why did I take such solace in sugar and junk food when she did not? Why, despite being a really happy and content kid with an idyllic upbringing, did I eat food when I wasn't hungry? What spurred me on to eat bag upon bag of sugary fizzy sweets even though they were making me fat?

The answer – I know now with the benefit of age – is simply that I am an emotional eater and Natalie is not. I will want to eat sweet stuff when I am bored, or when I feel anxious, under pressure or nervous – which was quite a lot of the time. Despite appearing to be outwardly confident, I've always been quite a shy and retiring person and I very rarely felt comfortable in my own skin. While I would act as if I were the life of the party, even as a teenager I preferred to stay in my bedroom rather than go out to the pub or a club. Although I was comfortable and happy around my own friends – and I'm fortunate to have always had lots of them – I felt embarrassed, shy and awkward if people I didn't know struck up a conversation with me, worrying that I would make an idiot of myself in some way. All this goes some way to explaining why, as a teenager, my friends and I would only go to one nightclub in Worthing called The Factory, where they played grunge music. It was more like a social club than anything else, and everyone knew each other, which created a certain air of safety. We went there almost every Saturday night for the duration of sixth form college. Where other teenagers turned to boozing to give themselves a bit of a spring in their step and some extra confidence, I turned to food (and a bit of booze). It made me feel good, and, best of all, unlike other people, I knew exactly what I was going to get with it. I thought I was in control.

Although my weight went up and down (at sixth form college I decided to only eat one packet of Quavers for lunch in a bid to lose some weight, and promptly went down to a size 10–12 from a size 16), I never stopped eating sugar.

'Young children have a palate that is predisposed to preferring sweet over sour or bitter, probably to protect them from eating poisonous food,' says clinical psychologist Dr Cecilia D'Felice. 'Because the first food we taste – our mother's milk – is incredibly naturally sweet, it follows that sweet becomes associated with feeling good, feeling satisfied, feeling cared for, feeling energised (there is a great deal of energy in sugar) and the associations then become made. Our palates do change as we mature, but our fondness for something sweet often remains because so much conditioning has been experienced.

'It's important to understand that sweet, like sour and bitter – are just symbols. It is the meaning you take from the foods that will determine your relationship with them.'

My relationship with food was just about to get a bit more entangled. At 18, I went off to university in Southampton. There, on the first day, I met Joe (not his real name), a graphic design student and skateboarder who was, conveniently, my neighbour in our halls of residence. He was my first serious boyfriend, and we ended up dating and living together for four years. I loved him massively. He didn't, however, help my sweet tooth.

When I went to university I was a small size 12; by the end of the first year I was a big size 14. Joe was a handsome, slim and active guy who'd spend his holidays snowboarding in the Czech Republic or skateboarding. He loved to DJ and would often get gigs in local clubs that would keep him out until 3 a.m. I'd go with him and we'd slurp free shots of flavoured vodka or spirits and mixers for hours on end. He seemed to be able to burn it off – me, not so much – although this was probably down to the fact that he exercised while I liked to sit on the sofa watching *Kilroy*.

In fact, whenever Joe went anywhere – out skating, to lectures, or to his part-time job – he'd frequently bring me back little tokens of his affection: often cans of Cherry Coca-Cola (my favourite) and those big 'Lucky Dip'-style bags of sweets that contained Love Hearts, Fizzers and Lollipops, which I'd proceed to munch throughout the afternoon and evening. We'd have plain chocolate digestives by the bed in a biscuit tin that I'd eat while watching telly at night or when I woke up. Joe wasn't a feeder and in no way set out to make me fat (although when we split up in 2000 I was a bit of a bloater), he was just buying me things that I enjoyed eating. But it's easy to see how love and food are so linked together.

Indeed, there's a large section in James Duigan's book about food and the emotional associations that come with it.

'For most of us, when we were growing up, sugary foods were used as a "reward" by our parents, grandparents and almost everyone else we knew,' he writes. 'When we felt sad because we'd scraped our knee, we were given sweets to cheer us up. As for birthdays, we'd get a huge cake, literally drenched in sugar to celebrate. Is it any wonder that by the time we reach our teens, we'd learnt to associate sugary foods with happy times and making ourselves feel better?'

Happiness, of course, isn't only a sense; something that is affected by external factors. No, being in a 'good mood' also comes down to the body's production of certain hormones, namely serotonin. And what helps the brain to produce more serotonin? Eating carbohydrates, especially sugar-rich ones.

'A serotonin deficiency causes serious clinical depression,' writes Professor Robert Lustig in his book *Fat Chance*. For the unfamiliar, Professor Lustig, an American paediatric endocrinologist, has transformed people's attitudes to sugar. Since it was posted online five years ago, a video of his lecture 'Sugar: The Bitter Truth' has had more than 4 million viewings. He continues. 'One way to increase serotonin production in the brain is to eat more carbohydrates – especially sugar. Over time however, more sugar is needed for the same effect... driving a vicious cycle of consumption to generate a meagre pleasure in the face of persistent unhappiness.'

Lustig believes that sugar is toxic and its consumption can lead to diseases such as diabetes. What's more, he says sugar is addictive. 'Not as addictive as tobacco or alcohol,' he told *The Sunday Times*, 'but if it's everywhere you can't get rid of it. The food industry knows when they add it to food you buy more.'

Can anyone else hear the sound of bells ringing? What Robert Lustig describes as a 'vicious cycle of consumption to generate meagre pleasure' certainly sounds familiar to me. While I've never been depressed and wouldn't describe myself as 'unhappy', certainly the mood swings and high levels of emotionality I've felt at times throughout my career have been nursed by foods. I realised that I had been unwittingly propagating a dependency that was now proving very hard to beat.

I wondered too, if my diet was contributing to my inability to cope with some of the stresses I was under at work. We've already learnt that refined foods make you stressed because they release sugar into the bloodstream too quickly, causing insulin spikes and altering our blood sugar. But perhaps this was at the root of my uneven moods – the fact that I could go to work grumpy, an hour later (after breakfast) feel amazing, another hour later feel overwhelmed (have a snack), then feel amazing, be at a loss before lunch and so on throughout the day until I collapsed into bed, sleeping fitfully before waking in the morning feeling far from refreshed and instantly craving something sweet.

There is a reference to this in James Duigan's book:

'The more uneven our blood sugar levels; the more uneven our moods become – we get hungry, angry and can't think clearly. We feel depressed and upset. Eating something high in sugar turns this back again – we feel happier, sharper and have more clarity – temporarily. But this pleasant spike soon gives way to an unpleasant crash. We feel panicky, wired... The more your blood sugar levels fluctuate, the more likely you are to react badly to life's stresses. And your reliance upon sugar becomes a trap.'

Stresses were something I was hoping to have few of when, about two months into my low-sugar plan, I went on holiday to Spain with a good female friend. We'd both been working flat out for the previous few months and were desperate to get away from it all. Single, stressed out from work and feeling my way through this new life without sugar had really taken it out of me. I craved a sunny break where the only certainty was that there'd be a lounger with my name on it out by the glittering blue sea every day. I suggested going to my parents' holiday apartment. The fact that it's near to a lovely fishing village often full of tall handsome Swedish men on boats had nothing to do with it.

I don't think, however, I'd adequately conveyed what I wanted from our week away to my travelling companion. While I was craving a sedate retreat, my friend was craving something with a bit more fiesta. Unsurprisingly, a couple of days in, I started to feel my abstinence from all things debaucherous – cocktails, ice cream and the like – was niggling her. Each time she offered to get me something from the beach bar and I abstained, instead reaching into my beach bag for a packet of oatcakes, I felt her grimace. I get it; your holiday buddy being virtuous makes you feel like you're somehow being 'bad'. But I wasn't setting out to make anyone feel anything; I'd just made my choices and was going to stick to them. I know what I'm like, I didn't want to have a few blow-out dinners, eat a few ice creams, get really drunk and spend the next day eating my bodyweight in simple carbs and chugging back orange juice by the gallon. Why would I ruin the last seven weeks for five days of that? I didn't want to go back to square one. There was a discussion one night at a bar where the whole 'life is too short to be so restrictive' line came out. But that was the whole point, life isn't short if you don't feel at your best.

Fair enough if it's something you can do little about, but my eating was something that was in my power to change, and I had to try my best to do so.

The trip ended up being rather more fraught than we'd both have liked. While we never came to blows, I felt – and perhaps it was just me – that there was something of a bad atmosphere. Like I'd fallen foul of some unspoken holiday code, 'thou must live unhealthily while on holiday'. From my side it wasn't a conscious thing – and I have to stress we are still very good friends – but perhaps we'd just succeeded in rubbing each other up the wrong way. It can happen on holidays, spending days side by side with someone you're not used to.

There was no doubt, however, that my food and drink conflicts were part of the niggle. And it was the first time I'd ever found something that's meant to be enjoyable, to be a source of conflict. I began to worry that sugar was the glue that held some of my relationships together and without it, perhaps, some of my much loved friendships would come unstuck. Sharing food and drink is, of course, a method of social bonding. We don't meet a friend for a drink because we're thirsty, we meet for a drink to see them. The Spain trip, coupled with the reactions of some of my female friends at the pub before I left (and my realisation that I no longer enjoyed being around drunk people) was making me rethink my whole social life.

As a feminist, I hate to point this out, but it is something I noticed. The people most bothered by my decision to quit crap foods and boozing were women. My guy friends couldn't give a damn. They'd have a beer if I was having a water, without even mentioning it. I began to wonder if women impart more value onto sugar, or if there's a biochemical reason that women are more susceptible to cravings for chocolate, cakes and other sweet treats. Is it just that these products have been marketed at us or is there something else at play? As far as I'm aware, men rarely egg each other on to eat another slice of chocolate cake, in the way that some women do (but I suppose some guys do it with drinking). Men wouldn't build a whole afternoon out around going for tea and cake, as I did with friends. Blokes just don't seem to give sweet food the same amount of attention as women do. Perhaps they reserve their competition and attentions for beer.

'Women don't have any biological or biochemical reason to eat more sugar than men,' says Ian Marber. 'There are no hormonal differences that make women want – or need – to eat more sweet foods. I think it simply comes down to advertising. After all, sugar cravings mainly come down to conditioning. We know this because sugar cravings are not a universal thing. People all over the world do not suffer from these feelings, it's a malady particular to us in the West. If we didn't eat sugar, we wouldn't crave it.'

I was fascinated. So, all the rather sexist viewpoints I'd always assumed were based in fact – you know, the whole 'women crave chocolate around the time they are getting their period' thing... it was actually rubbish, at least from a biochemical standpoint.

But even from an emotional standpoint, there is no reason why women should be more susceptible than men to the much-fabled 'sweet tooth' says clinical psychologist Dr Cecilia D'Felice.

'The symbol of femininity coupled with food is a very strong one in nearly all societies, because of the association made when mothers nurse their young,' she says. 'Thus women and food seem a natural partnership that then becomes hardwired into human consciousness. We will always have exceptions that prove the rule, but we can hardly say that men enjoy food or cooking less than women, they just don't have the same opportunity to express this nurturing or creative side of themselves.'

So, there you have it. Our obsession with sugar is probably mainly down to social conditioning – and marketing is a huge part of that.

Unsurprisingly, bearing in mind how much we consume, sugar is a massive industry with a lot of money behind it.

The likes of Coca-Cola, Kraft and Mars each make billions of pounds every year.

In 2013, *The Sunday Times* newspaper revealed that a draft proposal to cut the amount of sugar we eat had been put together by an expert panel at the World Health Organization (WHO). They came to this position after studying a report by Newcastle University's Professor Paula Moynihan that advised sugar intake should be reduced to prevent tooth decay. The WHO panel, however, were apparently mindful of the links between excessive sugar consumption and our ever-rising rates of obesity.

Their recommendation would be for individuals to halve the amount of sugar they consume. At present, the guidelines are that sugar intake should be no more than 10 per cent of your total energy intake. The new findings would mean reducing this to 5 per cent. The World Health Organization obviously has massive clout, and therefore, these recommendations are likely to be issued to governments, including our own here in the UK. This in turn could affect the food advice given out by the NHS and the 'traffic light' colour coding system displayed on the foods we buy. The knock-on effect is obvious: it could hit the big confectionery companies where it hurts, in their bank balances.

It's probably an understatement to say this wouldn't go down well.

A change in the official food guidelines would be a big

deal. As *The Sunday Times* notes, the WHO doesn't issue advice like this very often, indeed the last time it did so was in 2003 and it was met by much resistance from the all-powerful American Sugar Association that went on an aggressive campaign to 'expose the dubious nature' of the report and challenge the levels of funding given to the WHO by the American government.

Britain has its own sugar advocacy group, called Sugar Nutrition UK (which seems like an oxymoron bearing in mind many declare sugar to be an 'anti-nutrient' as it gives nothing and leaches out vitamins and minerals from the body, but I digress). Sugar Nutrition UK gets its money from the companies that make up Britain's sugar industry, including Associated British Foods, a company that *The Sunday Times* claims made £435 million profit from its sugar business in 2013. The World Sugar Research Organisation (WSRO) is also based in London and describes its mission on its website as being 'dedicated to encouraging a better appreciation of the direct and indirect contribution made by sugar to the nutrition, health and wellbeing of all the populations of the world'. Hmm. The WRSO is also funded by the sugar industry. Obviously, both groups are quick to argue that sugar is neither toxic, nor addictive.

For example, there is a statement on the Frequently Asked Questions section of Coca-Cola's website which declares that none of the ingredients in their drinks are addictive.

They state that people cannot develop an addiction because food and drinks aren't drugs, and that people often say they are 'addicted' to sugar or sweetened goods as a 'short-hand statement'. In other words, they have little scientific proof and just mean that it tastes good and they like to consume it on a regular basis.

Depending on the WHO's advice, it could be time for Coca-Cola to alter its website. And, out of interest, would Coca-Cola also deny caffeine is addictive? Because that's an ingredient in drinks produced by the Coca-Cola company too, and it's widely accepted that caffeine is highly addictive.

But I digress. While the effects of sugar are still the subject of much research and debate, what's becoming increasingly obvious are the dubious tactics employed by the sugar industry. Again, *The Sunday Times* refers to a 2013 speech by the director-general of the WHO, Margaret Chan 'who compared their tactics to those employed by the big tobacco firms, which for years dismissed scientific evidence that cigarettes were bad for health.'

"'It is not just Big Tobacco any more," she said. "Public health must also contend with Big Food, Big Soda and Big Alcohol. All of these industries fear regulation and protect themselves by using the same tactics. Research has documented these tactics well. They include front groups, lobbies, promises of self-regulation, lawsuits and industry-funded research that confuses the evidence and keeps the public in doubt.'"

'Research into food and nutrition in this country is partly funded by big business,' says Ian Marber. 'I liken it to a company that designs gas-guzzling cars working with the Government on lower emissions targets to help the environment. You have to ask yourself that while they may help reduce them, would they help eliminate them altogether?'

It's something to think about when you next tuck into that bag of chocolate.

Chapter Four

WHAT HAPPENS TO YOUR BODY?

Urban legend has it that it takes 21 days to break an old habit or make a new one. I remember a colleague telling me this when I was about a week into kicking sugar and I could have cried. Three weeks?! I wasn't sleeping properly, I was spotty and overweight, I felt upset and my digestion had gone into overdrive. And because I felt so unwell, I'd been living like a hermit. Two more weeks of enduring that felt like an eternity.

I went on the internet to seek solidarity through other people's experiences. Even three days in, some people were writing on forums that they felt 'amazing' and 'full of energy'. Huh? Who were these people? The only reason I dragged my bedraggled butt out of bed was to pay my mortgage, otherwise I'd have hibernated in my duvet cave for a good week or more.

But then I looked at it in a different way: in the scheme of your life, three weeks is really an impossibly short period of time to have to sacrifice in order to make the rest of your life happier and healthier.

Without going all 'New Age', I knew it was quite important to remember how rough I was feeling. It was kind of amazing that my body could tolerate all the rubbish I'd been putting into it, and terrifying how gross it felt now it was expunging it all. I made a decision that I'd never let my body get into this kind of desperate state of dependency again.

I've already told you that the jury is out as to whether sugar is addictive or not. Big brands like Coca-Cola – whose Spring 2014 ad slogan is, coincidentally, 'Open Happiness' – claim it is not addictive in the way that drugs, alcohol or tobacco are. As I'm fortunate enough never to have been addicted to any of those things I wouldn't know. It's certainly bloody hard to kick. I was shocked then, to find out that even eminent nutritionists such as Ian Marber don't believe sugar to be addictive.

> 'Sugar is pleasurable to eat,' he says. 'We have the taste receptors for sweet at the front of our tongues, so we are obviously biologically programmed, to a degree, to want to eat sweet things. It's a natural part of life.
>
> 'Of course, there is an emotional response to sugar too. People talk about being "addicted" to sugar, and in fact eating it does trigger a dopamine response in the brain [dopamine is a neurotransmitter that is released by some parts of the brain as a result of a rewarding experience, such as eating food, sex or taking drugs] but, to a lesser degree than we would

like to think. Saying "I'm addicted to sugar" is really saying "I like it a lot". While it is possible to have a biochemical dependency on the highs and the lows eating sugar can create, it's not really possible to be addicted to sugar itself.

'Our culture creates a guilt around eating sweet things. People tend to want to be able to "blame" their taste for sugar on something else – like it being genetic or the fact that they're "addicted". There's nothing wrong with liking something.

'It's not a modern phenomenon either. People ate High Tea in Victorian times, they had sweet fancies in Roman times. Processed food is modern, but otherwise we have always eaten sugar because it tastes nice and it makes us feel good, not because of an "addiction".'

Okay, so if it's not addictive from a physiological perspective, is sugar addictive from an emotional standpoint? I asked clinical psychologist Dr Cecilia D'Felice:

'Something is only going to be emotionally addictive if the individual makes it so,' she says. 'If the symbol of sugar has been set up in your mind to be the enemy; then it will become the enemy. Remember that all symbols – including sugar – are inherently neutral until meaning is projected into them. For one person, sugar may be loaded with meaning, such as it is delicious, fun, enjoyable, healthy and makes you feel good. For another, the symbol of sugar could be loaded with an opposite set of values, such as it is bad, fattening, unhealthy, gives you bad skin...

'There was a time when sugar was only found in unrefined fruits, nuts and honey. Then it was not considered anything other than a wonderful gift. With refining it came a different association with sugar. It was made by slaves. That's going to make anyone feel guilty about consuming it.

'An idea that is shared, grows in strength. If your family, group of friends or society see sugar as a bad thing, you are likely to see it as a bad thing too. If you don't, then sugar may not be seen as the enemy, but just a normal and enjoyable part of your diet.'

In other words, sugar can be thought of as emotionally addictive if we have conditioned ourselves into putting meaning on to it.

Phew, it's all a bit complex. But I know I am guilty of seeing something as innocuous and unemotional as a slab of combined sugar and fat – in other words, chocolate – as in some way meaningful. From Joe bringing me bags of sweets to getting a quarter of sherbet pips at the sweet shop for an after-school treat on a Friday afternoon, sugar has always been loaded with emotions for me – and probably most of us in the Western world.

Also, regardless of what Ian or Cecilia say, I felt an acute physical withdrawal when I stopped eating it. Bona fide feelings of illness – headaches, weakness, interrupted sleep, spots and all the other things I have already documented. If gambling and shopping (both emotional behaviours rather than physical ones) are seen as addictions then why isn't sugar?

Here's what James Duigan has to say about it in his *Clean and Lean Diet* book.

'Food should be enjoyed when you're relaxed and happy. It's not something that should stir up feelings of shame, guilt or despair. When you view food as the "enemy", you'll get stuck in that all-too-common cycle of deprivation and reward – the reward being a binge on fatty sugary foods that give a quick fleeting high followed by a feeling of sickness, tiredness and, ultimately, guilt and shame. Then the cycle of deprivation will happen again.'

So, is there any truth in the whole 21-days-to-make-or-break-a-habit thing? A bit of researching revealed to me that it's a completely empirical statement, in other words it's never been proven in a clinical setting. Hmmmm. Evidence suggests that new habits are easier to form than to break and, if you repeat an action often enough, the brain will create new pathways and it will become natural. Whether that takes 21 days or not is down to each individual's brain and personality.

Now comes the hard part: breaking a habit. Research shows that while worn-in pathways weaken when you stop doing something – eating a chocolate digestive when you wake up, for example – they never go away and can be re-activated with the smallest amount of encouragement.

In other words, you have to be strict with yourself if you are serious about quitting something you enjoy.

The only way I got through those first few difficult weeks of change was to keep my eyes on the prize. And the prize was a healthier, slimmer, happier me. Now, I am not good at this. Any of my friends will tell you that positive mental attitude has never been one of my strong points, but it was absolutely essential to getting over this three-week hump. And that's when the good stuff started to happen.

Ian Marber has already told us what goes on in our bodies when we stop eating sugar after eating a lot of it. Your blood glucose levels go haywire, your protein levels can be low and your adrenal glands have to work hard, creating feelings of extreme highs and lows. The bacteria in your intestines are often out of balance, which makes you tired and can play havoc with your digestion. Because excessive sugar intake depletes the body's store of magnesium and B-vitamins (they are responsible for getting energy from food and maintaining healthy brain functions and mental clarity) you'll feel mentally 'foggy'. I likened the feeling to someone having removed my brain and replaced it with water.

However long these feelings last for you – and for me it was about ten days – once they're gone they're gone and, as Yazz put it so wonderfully back in 1988, 'The Only Way Is Up'.

Some changes became obvious almost immediately, while others took longer to manifest. Below, I'll outline all the things that I noticed in the order that I noticed them.

ONE WEEK – digestion overdrive

I don't want to talk too much about poop. It's not nice. But, as my friend Lee Mullins, Director of Personal Training at James Duigan's Bodyism gym says, people these days just don't poo enough. It's true. There are no hard and fast rules about how many times you should go per day but – sorry for the sentence that's coming next – apparently it's the consistency that counts. The week before I revamped my diet, I was probably going once a day, sometimes once every couple of days. Then all of a sudden I was going three times a day. It's not rocket science. I was obviously eating lots more vegetables and much less processed food that tends to hang around in your guts for longer. If you want to try and get rid of bloating, help your body get rid of waste quickly rather than let it sit there fermenting in your tummy.

TWO WEEKS – clearer eyes

I've already spoken about receiving compliments on my eyes. Out of the blue, colleagues commented that they looked either 'brighter', 'clearer' or 'twinkly'. It was strange, as having clearer eyes wasn't something I ever noticed, but after two different people had said it to me I decided to investigate why this could be. I found out that when your liver is under stress, trying to eliminate a lot of waste from the body (an excess of sugar, fat and the like) it can cause the whites of your eyes to become slightly yellow – it's called icterus. While my eyes weren't ever noticeably yellow, perhaps giving my liver less work to do made them appear clearer. The dark circles under my eyes that had plagued me for a good few years also disappeared after about three weeks, probably because of the improvements in my sleep.

THREE WEEKS – better sleep

While I slept terribly during the first few days of cutting down on sugar, my quality of kip was another thing that improved fairly rapidly when I gave it up. For about six months before I decided to come off sugar I'd been suffering bouts of mid-sleep insomnia. As ever, I would drop off easily, and was asleep within about a minute of deciding I wanted to sleep. Around 3 a.m., however (after about three and a half hours of shut-eye), I'd wake up, immediately wired. No matter how hard I tried – using pillow sprays, taking the herbal sleeping tablet valerian, wearing ear plugs, not drinking water in the hours before going to bed and turning off all external stimulants such as my phone and laptop – I still woke up. Worst of all, I stayed awake for a good couple of hours, fretting about how tired I would be at work the next day. Anyone who has ever had insomnia knows how debilitating it is, and so-called 'sleep-maintenance insomnia' (the professional term for waking in the middle of the night) is the most commonly reported kind. A poor quality of sleep is linked to many things, and blood sugar spikes throughout the day is just one of them.

When we are asleep our brain still needs a constant supply of energy. Over time, if we eat a high sugar diet our body gets used to using sugar as its main energy source. It struggles to keep a constant supply of glucose (sugar) for our brain to use efficiently because of the spikes and crashes in blood sugar levels that are associated with a high sugar diet. In the day we mostly compensate by eating more sugar when our levels drop, but at night the body relies on its own mechanisms to increase the levels if they fall too low. Our adrenal glands produce a hormone called cortisol; one of its functions is to control how the body makes energy. If there's not enough glucose, our cortisol helps to convert fats and proteins into glucose by a process called gluconeogenesis. However, cortisol production can become impaired over time as unbalanced blood sugar levels places the body under stress. Therefore, when our blood sugar levels drop at night but we don't provide the quick fuel the body has been accustomed to (sugar!) and our adrenals are not producing cortisol efficiently to make the glucose from other sources, adrenaline can kick in. This 'fight or flight' response happens so the body can somehow get it's blood glucose levels back up but the result is that you wake up.

While I was going through what I rather melodramatically call 'my withdrawal' I felt this acutely. Not only did I have problems going to sleep – which was a first – but my sleep was disrupted when I did finally drift off. I was hot and clammy but also woke several times feeling hugely anxious and emotional for no reason, worrying, then going back to a very light, highly aware type of slumber. It was completely exhausting. While it was worse in week one, by week two things began improving and by week three I was collapsing into bed at the end of the day and sleeping right the way through. It felt like a miracle.

Of course it wasn't really a miracle, it's all down to science. Ian Marber puts it simply.

'People who don't have sugar highs and lows throughout the day will sleep better.'

D'oh.

FOUR WEEKS – getting lighter

I like to think I am not vain. Yet I get my hair highlighted every six weeks, have my eyebrows threaded, get waxed, have facials, wear make-up, exercise, blah blah blah. So, while I could say that my health was my primary motivation for giving up sugar, it wouldn't be true – my weight took equal priority. But I have never been a scales obsessive. To me, numbers on a dial are irrelevant; we all know if we are too heavy. As a bit of a clothes horse, I always go by how my favourite items feel when I slip them on in the morning.

In May 2012 I bought an expensive dress from Dolce & Gabbana for my birthday party, in a size 16. Now there is nothing wrong with being a size 16 – it's the UK's average dress size, and, being tall (I'm 5′ 10″), I could carry it off, to a certain degree. Yet I really didn't want to be a size 16 and, what's more, I haven't always been. In my late teens I was a size 12, and I wanted to be that way again. Looking podgy made me unhappy, but more importantly, being podgy was unhealthy. We all know being overweight puts extra strain on your heart (and I already had a genetic heart defect) and other organs, it increases your blood pressure, can lead to type 2 diabetes and other health issues and puts extra strain on your joints. Running was hard work and I kept getting injured – probably because I was too heavy to run. My cycle route to and from work has some pretty steep hills in it and by the time I got anywhere I was often red faced. 'That bloody Pashley bicycle is so heavy,' I'd say to anyone who'd listen when I got into the office, and it was, especially with my bag in the front basket. 'And,' I'd continue, 'it only has five gears.' While both of these points were true, I was excluding the fact that it was also hard work pushing myself up those hills of a morning.

While I've always had slim arms and legs, a diet high in refined sugars, alcohol and processed foods will cause your body to store weight on the thighs, hips, tummy, waist and back. Tick tick tick tick tick.

In short, I wanted to lose the extra pounds. But I've never been someone for whom weight just falls off. Many of my colleagues would arrive at their desks in the mornings munching on a pain au chocolat washed down with a huge café latte and not put on a pound. I, however, only had to look at a ham and cheese baguette to feel my jeans tighten. When I did put on weight it took me a long time to lose it (this, coincidentally, is another indicator of having a degree of insulin resistance).

I didn't, however, want to be miserable losing weight. I didn't want to consume lots of man-made foods or artificial drinks, which are ultimately unsatisfying. If I did that, I knew I wouldn't stick to it. That meant no points, no coloured days, no 'sins', weigh-ins or other – to my mind – ultimately unsustainable ways of dropping pounds. While they may work for some people, organised eating plans whereby someone tells you what to do on a certain day have never been my bag. And that was what I found about going low sugar, it was so easy to sustain. But, like anything, you have to want to do it. The hardest part was truly accepting that you value the long-term things – namely your health and appearance – over the short-term things like eating processed foods, lots of fruit and simple carbohydrates, and drinking alcohol.

It was as I passed the four-week marker that I started receiving a lot of compliments. While I'd lost weight from all over my body, it was from around my tummy and sides that I noticed it first. Don't get me wrong, I was still a long way from having a flat tummy, but it was certainly flatter – as I would expect after I'd cut out lots of the foods I previously enjoyed. My clothes felt looser and I'd let my belt in a notch. As the weeks progressed, the weight kept steadily falling off. I lost track of how many people commented on it. My bingo wings disappeared, my bum felt a bit less wobbly. My boobs, too, shrank – indeed this was one of the first things an ex-boyfriend commented on when he saw me in the street (that kind of comment explains why he's an ex). In fact, instead of 'weight-loss', 'shrinkage' would be a good way to describe the whole process. Since summer 2012, I have gone down from a size 16 to a size 10–12. Had someone told me this at the beginning, I would totally have taken that.

FOUR WEEKS – better skin

Being single does have its benefits. Sleeping alone meant that I was free to slather my face in antiseptic cream before hitting the hay. I daubed great big gelatinous white blobs of the stuff over any pimples that had sprung up during the day. As well as covering my jawline – where the majority of the little blighters had taken up residence – the cream simultaneously covered my bed linen and pillowcases. So far, so unsexy. In the mornings, before I'd even opened my eyes I would feel my face to see if I'd had a new breakout overnight. Suddenly getting bad skin in my thirties after previously having a good complexion was both mystifying and upsetting.

Aside from the acne, my skin had become dull. In the mornings I'd get up, bound into the bathroom to perform my ablutions and be greeted by a blotchy grey-faced lady (half covered in spot cream) staring back at me. I used expensive face scrubs to try and slough off any dead skin cells, but after 30 minutes or so, when the rosiness from the improved circulation had died down, I didn't look too different. Perplexing.

This too was getting me down: every time I so much as showed my pale face to the sun, I'd get a patch of pigmentation pop up, either on my forehead or on my top lip. The dreaded hormone moustache, as my friend Olivia calls it. While any woman who's ever been pregnant or on a form of hormonal birth control will recognise the pigmentation issue, I was neither of those things. I couldn't understand it.

I'd tried treating my skin from the outside – as well as the nightly spot cream adventures my job meant I'd been able to try regular courses of intensive facials from some of the best names in the business. Nothing made any lasting difference.

As getting spots around your jawline is often related to a hormonal issue, I don't suppose it would.

Then there were the dreaded 'fine lines and wrinkles' so beloved of anti-ageing cream companies. Despite working in the industry, I've spent years trying not to feel the pressure to conform to some sort of ever-youthful ideal. After finding out I had a heart condition at 27, a large part of me worried that I wasn't going to get to the stage of actually getting any wrinkles, anyhow. But then in a spectacular case of 'be careful what you wish for', within a couple of years I had them in abundance. While they obviously didn't appear 'overnight', I began noticing something of a glut of them, mainly underneath my eyes and deeper ones across my forehead. Nothing really had changed to bring about this sudden manifestation. Yes, I was getting older, but my skin wasn't dry, I hadn't been out in the sun without wearing a sunscreen with a decent SPF and I was still drinking a litre and a half of water every day.

My elaborate cleansing and moisturising routine wasn't doing anything to help either. No creams – no matter how expensive – can make your wrinkles disappear. Many are great at hydrating and plumping up the skin, which makes any wrinkles look better or even reduced, but disappear? Give me a break. The only things that can do that are injectable fillers, Botox or a facelift, and I wasn't ready for that.

So I continued doing what I was doing and found solace in a good foundation by Yves Saint Laurent. Although it can't work wonders on wrinkles, make-up can cover a multitude of sins.

I was curious though, as to what was causing my skin to look so, well, crap, so quickly.

Then I reduced my sugar intake. Within a month my spots had gone. Sure, there were red marks and scars where the ones I'd had were healing, but for the first time in years, new ones weren't arriving on an almost daily basis. My skin was still congested and when I went to Spain, I got some pigmentation, but as the months went by and I went abroad to other sunny places, I stopped getting it so badly. I don't want to brag, but friends said my skin looked glowing or healthy – comments I never would have received two years ago. Curious, I asked former A&E medic, turned cosmetic doctor, Mica Engel of London's Waterhouse Young Clinic what happens to our faces when we eat a lot of junk. What she told me was fascinating:

'The main theory now to explain why we age revolves around a so-called tripod of things: free radicals, sun damage and glycation' she says.

'Our skin starts ageing when we're 25. Before that age we have fast cell renewal that gives us our doughy peachy complexions. After 25, everything starts to slow down; in ancient times, people didn't live much past 30, so it didn't matter if things started to wear out. Now of course, we live until we are 80 or 90 and our biology hasn't caught up.

'But, at 25, the body starts to lose its ability to deal with sun damage, free radicals and glycation.

'Let me explain what these things actually mean. Glycation is when excess glucose from the blood-stream binds to the skin's "youth proteins" (the col-lagen and elastin that makes youthful complexions appear so plump and doughy) and instead turns them brittle and stiff. It effectively "caramelises" the surface of the cells, meaning collagen and elastin fibres in the skin can no longer perform their most important roles – namely cell division and tissue renewal. Without this, wrinkles and saggy skin will appear on the face prematurely. Over time, the problem magnifies. The by-products of glycation accumulate in the body and skin constantly appears dull and aged.

'While it is a natural ageing response, some lifestyle factors such as eating a diet high in sugar or cooking food until it burns or chars (like under a grill or on a barbecue) accelerates the process of glycation. That's why steaming food or eating it raw is better for you.

'Next, let's take free radicals. These unstable molecules are a natural by-product of the body processing the nutrients from the food we eat and drink. If you eat lots of fat and sugar, which are hard for the liver to break down, the metabolism has to ramp up a gear to process it and you have more unstable free radicals floating around. These molecules then attach to something else to be neutralised, and they attach to collagen in the skin and break it down.

'Lastly, sun damage. We have a whole generation who were exposed to harmful UVA and UVB rays through going on sunbeds. They have the skin quality of a 40- or 50-year-old, yet they're in their twenties. They have wrinkles, pigmentation, they look like they have old skin. About 80 per cent of our sun damage is done before we reach the age of 25. Simply using sun block during your teenage years is a massive investment in your skin for later down the line.'

While our skin may start ageing at 25, Mica is quick to point out that we shouldn't start seeing the *signs* of ageing – fine wrinkles, pigmentation, dull blotchy skin, a lack of elasticity – until we are about 35. Anything before that is deemed 'premature ageing'.

'What we eat definitely shows in our face. Excessively high blood sugar causes the body to raise its production of insulin,' she says. 'Both of these processes cause "micro-inflammation" in the cells, which is now thought to increase the rate at which our skin ages.

'Your skin is your biggest organ and it is showing you how your body is suffering on the inside. This micro-inflammation I've been talking about shows on the skin as pigmentation, redness, broken veins, spots. Perhaps you've noticed your skin has started to lose elasticity, often the jawline is the first place that becomes slack. Also, the texture of your skin starts to change; you get an uneven complexion, fine wrinkles, which lead to deeper wrinkles as the time goes on, dilated pores. It's a whole process.'

This is not just anecdotal research. In 2011, scientists from Holland's Leiden University Medical Center and Unilever's R&D centre measured the blood sugar levels of 600 people to see if there was indeed a direct link between how much sugar circulates in the blood and how old a person looks. Their findings show that (even taking into consideration other factors such as whether a person smokes), those with high blood sugar levels looked up to one-third older than those at the lower end of the scale.

Interestingly, Mica agrees that it is pointless to spend money on an anti-ageing regime or treatments if you are not going to tackle what is going on inside your body.

'Taking exercise and being careful with your diet is fundamental in ageing well,' she says. 'It's the first thing you should change if you are really concerned about ageing. I know it seems so simple, but just changing those things really makes so much difference. Supplements – such as vitamin D in the winter, or possibly vitamin A and E – will eventually have their place, but it's most important to get your food intake right.'

If you're feeling a little bleak at the prospect of what all those ice creams could have done to your complexion, fear not.

'You can reverse much of the damage that gets done once you have altered your diet to try and slow down the process,' Mica says. 'See a dermatologist or a cosmetic doctor to try and diagnose the type of pigmentation or acne you are suffering from. There are lots of treatments you can have to improve the appearance of your skin. Pigmentation can be eliminated with creams, the skin's texture can be improved with treatments including alpha-hydroxy acids, which are very good at promoting cell renewal. It's never too late to start taking care of yourself. If your skin is good on the outside, the inside will be good too.'

Still not convinced? Earlier this year the *Mail on Sunday* ran an interview with Victoria Beckham's Beverly Hills dermatologist Dr Henry Lancer to find out how she had transformed her skin from being prone to acne to the clear complexion we see now. He said:

'Victoria Beckham is a natural beauty. She's an incredible health nut – she watches her diet, her exercise, she sort of leads an ideal healthy life.

'She suffered badly from acne but [her skin now] is totally self resolved. She's an example of self-discipline. I always advise acne patients to modify their diets so they have no dairy intake, no caffeine intake, and next to no sugar.

'This means their carbohydrate intake has to be under 20 per cent of their calorific intake. I'm the only skin doctor who she's ever seen, so trust me on this one.'

SIX WEEKS – better moods

Many journalists are argumentative so-and-sos. It's almost part of the job description. While I'm not one to hold a grudge or bear anyone ill will for a prolonged period of time, I have always been quick to anger and, thankfully, quick to calm down. Although my anger is almost always directed at a situation or a thing rather than a person (I'm not one of those shouty types), over the past few years, I've found myself losing my temper more quickly at the smallest of things. I've always had a tendency to dissolve into tears when I get angry or frustrated, but it was happening more and more frequently. Although this is not exclusively down to my consumption of sugar, because of course, lots of things contribute to mood swings, including tiredness and stress levels (both of which are also affected by sugar, but I digress), there's plenty of evidence that sugar makes the problems worse.

Indeed, earlier in the book I've written about how consuming sugar – or foods that quickly turn to sugar inside the body – doesn't help you deal with stress (as we often imagine it does), but actually makes you feel more wired and less able to deal with difficult situations. It kind of flies in the face of the whole 'had a bad day? Have a bar of chocolate' legend that many of us have adopted as we've aged.

There is also scientific evidence that refined sugars – the types that are in processed food and drinks or added to food – perpetuate a cycle of mood swings. Take my example. A few years ago, at work on Fridays we'd have a cake to celebrate the end of the week. I know it sounds ridiculous now, but it was something of a tradition. Someone would go to the shop and buy a chocolate fudge cake. Of course, back then I would have a lovely piece of this chocolate cake and feel amazing for about 45 minutes. Then I'd start feeling rubbish – we used to call it 'the food coma'. I felt tired, cranky, in need of another bit of cake to give me the brainpower I needed to finish writing the headlines in the section I edited... So, perhaps I'd have another small sliver, 'just the tiniest of slices'. Hurrah, I felt good again, thank goodness I indulged. But then an hour later I felt even worse. This was my cue to venture down to the canteen and buy a can of diet fizzy drink to boost my energy and see me through until home time. Before I knew it, I'd polished off an extra 600 calories just sitting at my desk.

It's easy to see how living this way becomes a trap. As your blood sugar levels spike and slump, so do your emotions. If I hadn't had the first piece of cake, I wouldn't have had the second or the can of fizzy drink.

While I was going through the acute withdrawal phase from sugar, an improvement in moods was not something I noticed. If anything, I had a foul temper, probably because the rest of my system was so unbalanced. However, within about six weeks I started to feel generally more laid back and the pattern continued.

Unless, that is, my companion decides to speak on his work mobile phone for the duration of a 90-minute car journey to a 'special' non-work day out of London; turning the sat-nav down so it doesn't interrupt his chat, which results in my driving the wrong way down a one-way country lane and having to do an Austin Powers-style 12-point turn to the accompaniment of other cars horns. True story. On *those* occasions, I still have the propensity to completely lose my shit, pardon my French.

TWO MONTHS – a big boost in energy

I got the memo. Other people who change their diet and begin going low sugar claim to experience a huge surge in energy after just a few hours. This didn't happen to me. For the first few weeks after changing my eating habits, I just felt very tired. While I've never been a napper or someone who sleeps in the day, I would spend the second half of the day looking forward to the time I could clamber into bed. Again, this could be down to a number of things, firstly that my heart condition necessitates I take a beta blocker every day to make my heart beat slowly, which doesn't exactly cause you to scamper out of bed in the morning. My hours at work probably didn't help a great deal either.

While I'd always found the energy to go to the gym at 6.45 a.m. before starting work, I started to struggle and skip a few sessions. I began to only cycle one way to work, leaving my bike there overnight and cycling home the next evening. Perhaps it won't be like this for you, but for the first few weeks, physical exertion felt like a bit of an effort.

I was pretty rigidly sticking to my eating plan though, which was my priority. Then, one week at the end of summer it was as if a switch was flicked. In Chapter Two, Ian Marber likens going low sugar to changing over fuel tanks. You're going from one easily accessible form of energy – sugar – to another less accessible one. To continue his analogy, I felt as if I'd had a fuel injection. My colleague Emma and I recruited her old personal trainer Holly Pannett to come and train us one lunchtime a week outside in the beautiful Kensington Gardens, opposite our office. Holly's trained all manner of models and celebrities, and then she had Emma and I, huffing and puffing our way through press-ups in what is effectively Kate Middleton's back garden. Glamorous we were not.

But, to use a phrase beloved of 1960s hippies, I felt as if I had my groove back. Holly is also a nutritionist so, between tricep dips on a log, I breathlessly told her about my new eating regime. She gave me tips and tricks, suggested recipes (you can read more of these in Chapter Six) and provided inspiration. Holly is a moderate and always encouraged me to have fun while being healthy: 'you can do both' she would say. She was right. Together we began working on the areas I wanted to target – namely the excess weight around my waist, which had gradually been accumulating, particularly over the last few years of stressful working.

'There's a direct relationship between sugar and levels of the stress hormone cortisol,' she said. 'Cortisol has been shown to increase central fat distribution – in other words the chubby bits around your middle. By limiting your sugar intake you will quickly target this area.'

She was right. Within four months, I'd dropped over a stone and a half and the sleepy feeling that had been punctuating my afternoons had all but disappeared. Although I'm never going to be someone who bounds out of bed in the morning (unless there's a new dress waiting to be put on), when I was up and about I felt like a new person. Which I was becoming, slowly.

TWO MONTHS – bring on the wellness

I've never been a sickly person. Aside from a bout of dysentery I contracted after ill-advisedly swallowing some river water at Tonlé Sap in Cambodia a couple of years ago, I'm very rarely ill. However, I did suffer with repeated sore throats.

They started in 2008. I hadn't had tonsillitis since I was at school, but, as November rolled around I came down with a viral case of it. No sooner had I got rid of it than it returned again in January and again in April. Most of us have had tonsillitis at some stage or another, but it's easy to forget how debilitating it can be to have a temperature, throbbing headache and a throat that feels like it's lined with razor blades. Unfortunately, it was to become my norm. For four years I got tonsillitis three, four or even five times a year. Sometimes it was bacterial and I'd receive antibiotics. In fact, I was given a pre-emptive prescription of amoxicillin to take with me when I went on holiday in case it flared up. It happened in winter and summer, when I was stressed and when I wasn't. Often, there seemed to be no obvious cause and I just had to wait for my body to eliminate it. I didn't get colds, headaches, stomach bugs or flu, but it was always just this. It got so bad the doctor told me my tonsils had become scarred and that could be why I kept getting it. In 2012, as my glands were swollen, I was sent to a throat specialist for the obligatory camera up the nose and down the throat scenario. Thankfully there was nothing out of the ordinary.

Yet it was a mystery. I considered having my tonsils taken out, but was advised against it as it's quite a big operation when you're an adult. So that was that, I just had to accept that having a sore throat was my normal.

But then as quickly as my sore throats came on, they disappeared. I haven't had a bout since November 2012, six months after I gave up sugar. Are the two things linked? Ian Marber thinks so.

'Eating a diet rich in all types of sugars would have an effect on your immune system for two reasons.' Ian says. 'Firstly, it would deplete your magnesium stores and magnesium is responsible for maintaining a healthy immune system. Magnesium is also required, in its simplest form, as a glucose carrier. In order for glucose to get into the body's cells and be stored, it requires magnesium. If the body is always trying to deal with excess glucose, you are dipping into your magnesium stores constantly, which can suppress the production of white blood cells (the cells that fight off disease and bacteria). Additionally, if the body suffers dips in glucose, it produces adrenaline. Adrenaline also depletes magnesium levels.

'Secondly, eating sugars encourages fermentation in the gut, which can reduce the number of probiotics [probiotics are bacteria that can help support the immune system]. This is another reason you'd get coughs and colds.'

Quit refined sugar, become a bionic woman. Do you need a better reason?

EIGHT MONTHS – so long painful periods

I've already given you a potted history of my gynaecological issues (sorry about that). After quitting sugar I found out I had polycystic ovarian syndrome (PCOS) – a condition whereby your ovaries have harmless cysts on them. It's the most common gynaecological problem, with an estimated one in five women suffering from it. It was picked up during a routine ultrasound for something else, as I'd never really had any cause to think I had it.

But looking back at it now, all the signs were there. Since my early twenties, I'd always suffered with quite irregular and painful periods. They didn't affect my life, I still did everything that I would normally do, but they did get me down a bit.

When I went low sugar, I didn't know I had PCOS so I wasn't looking for any miracle cures. But whaddayaknow,

I got some anyhow. Within a matter of months, my periods had regulated themselves. They also became much less painful, and, for the first time in years I didn't need to sit on the sofa with a hot water bottle for a couple of nights a month.

I know now that researchers believe that many women with PCOS produce too much insulin – the hormone that controls how we use or store sugar in our bodies – and therefore advise women with the condition to eat less sugar because it exacerbates the symptoms.

But even if you don't have PCOS, significantly reducing your sugar intake can benefit your periods. Ian explains why.

'Magnesium is involved in muscle release and muscle contraction. In the simplest of terms, calcium contracts the muscle, magnesium releases it. If you suffer painful periods, it could be because you have used up some of your magnesium reserves.'

All of these were things I experienced within a few months of ditching the sweets I used to adore so much. While I had read other people's testimonies of how amazing they felt and how vibrant they looked after giving up the white stuff, I never really expected all this to happen to me. I'll admit it, a large part of me thought them to be evangelists, zealots with an agenda. But they were right. Too much sugar really does wreck your body from the inside out.

But even after seeing all those changes, I still thought about sugar a lot of the time. I still found myself leering longingly into other people's shopping baskets with their glazed doughnuts and their boxes of Frosties and their packets of chocolate chip shortbread. While I no longer felt compelled to wrestle them to the ground in the middle of the confectionery aisle and stuff squares of Green & Black's mint-filled dark chocolate into my mouth, I did still occasionally feel deprived. While I wasn't sure if it would ever go away, I had it under control. Just.

So, are you eating too much sugar? How would you even know? I asked Ian Marber to tell me what he'd expect to see in a patient who was consuming too much of the white stuff. Here, in no particular order, are some of the symptoms he looks out for:

- Fatigue
- Cravings
- A coating on the tongue
- Flatulence (because food would be fermenting in the gut)
- Poor skin quality or shiny skin
- Difficulty losing weight/weight stored around the middle
- Poor sleep
- Bad moods or quick to anger
- Muscle cramps
- Period pains

Interestingly, Ian also points out that being fat or thin is neither here nor there when it comes to sugar dependencies.

'Being thin and eating a lot of sugar doesn't mean you've "got away with it". It doesn't make it "okay". In fact, eating bad food and not putting on weight is not a marvellous thing because gaining weight and not feeling great is a wonderful way of changing behaviours. It's interesting that we still think of being thin as a licence to do what you like. It really isn't.'

Convinced? Want to join the low-sugar revolution. It's easy when you know how, and that's exactly what I'll show you in Chapter Five.

Chapter Five

HOW TO GO LOW SUGAR

By now, you've either been completely swayed to quit the white stuff or hideously put off, but as you're still reading, I'm imagining it's the former. I hope so.

I don't have any vested interests in telling you to overhaul your diet. If you're happy with what you eat and don't want to change, then no problem, carry on with your life.

But perhaps reading my story has rung a few bells with you. Maybe you'd like to target that bit of excess weight you're storing around your tummy. Perhaps you've been suffering with mood swings and bad sleep and spots and all the other things we write off and put down to some amorphous ill… 'Stress', for example. 'Being run down', or, my old personal favourite 'just not feeling right'.

Perhaps you've felt like this for a long time – maybe even years – but know this: it's not how you are meant to feel.

Three years ago, it would have been impossible for me to imagine writing this book. I wouldn't have envisaged I could stick to anything that I believed 'limited my options'. Yet I have, and you can too.

Be under no illusions, at the beginning it's going to feel hard. Yet, as the days go by – and we are talking days not months or years – living low sugar will become second nature to you. You'll still be able to go out for dinner, grab food on the go and enjoy an evening out with friends. But your choices will change. In fact, many things about you will change. You will sleep better, you'll be trimmer and more energetic and you'll have less cravings and mood swings. You'll get ill less often. Importantly, your whole idea of what constitutes a 'reward' or a 'treat' will alter.

For example, I no longer see drinking half a bottle of wine after work as a treat. A rotten night's sleep and the resultant fuzzy head the next morning isn't my idea of a good time. I work a lot; I want to maximise my time off, wake up, get out of bed and feel ready for the day ahead. When I used to drink more, I would often skip dinner and instead snack while I was out or eat some toast when I got in. The next day, waking up with a woolly head, I was often both famished and in need of quick energy so would crave an unhealthy breakfast. While I wouldn't succumb, the thought of buying a McDonald's Sausage and Egg McMuffin on the way into work often loomed large. The day would continue with my eating high-carbohydrate, sugar-rich foods to give me enough energy to see me through until I could go home and celebrate having made it through with a takeaway Indian meal or something similar. Looking at it as a whole, those 'couple of large glasses' of wine after work don't seem like such a harmless treat anymore.

Not drinking very often doesn't affect my social life, and it doesn't need to affect yours. Take last night for example. I went for dinner with a great friend, also called Nicole. We went to see a film at the cinema, then on to a stir-fry place and had a feast – chicken and cashew nut curry, some stir-fry greens, brown rice – there was lots of food. The other Nicole had a glass of white wine; I did not. It didn't ruin my evening, it didn't ruin hers. In fact it wasn't even mentioned by either of us. See? It's really pretty easy. It just comes down to the choices you make.

If you're ready to 'choose to change' then there's no reason why doing what I've done won't bring the same life-changing experiences for you as it did for me.

So, in this chapter, I am going to show you how you can go low sugar in a step-by-step way. As ever, if you have any medical problems, are overweight, or taking any form of medication or are seeing your doctor for any reason, or you are in any way unsure whether or not you should cut out sugar, you should make an appointment to go and see your GP or specialist who can advise you on the right way to implement changes into your diet.

But firstly, and most importantly, let's go back over what actually constitutes 'sugar' in the first place.

STEP 1. KNOW YOUR SUGARS

'There are effectively four types of sugar,' says nutritionist Ian Marber. Let me explain this further.

Added sugar or refined sugar

This is either the spoonful you add to your morning tea, or the six teaspoons that are found in a can of Coca-Cola. It's present in almost all processed foods, and processed foods are easy to identify. Basically, they bear little or no resemblance to their original ingredients. For example, shop-bought biscuits look little or nothing like their ingredients did in their natural state. Nutritionists are very concerned about the addition of fructose (a fruit sugar)to the majority of ready-made things that we buy in a highly processed form.

Fructose is bad because, unlike the other sugars, our body doesn't produce a hormonal response to this sugar (as it does with insulin for other sugars) to remove it from our bloodstream. Instead, the body sends fructose straight to the liver to deal with it. 'When the liver gets overwhelmed,' says Ian, 'it begins converting fructose to liver fat, which can cause fatty liver disease. Nowadays, this is becoming increasingly common and it ups our chances of developing a degree of insulin resistance, thickened arteries and heart disease.'

Fructose also suppresses the body's production of the hormone leptin, which tells you when you're full. In other words, you can never get enough of it.

Foods that naturally contain high amounts of sugars that you don't want

While not 'unhealthy', many fruits do contain high amounts of sugar – the exception are dark berries that are low GI (see below). Also wine, fruit juices and smoothies.

Foods that quickly convert to sugar in the body

These are easily identifiable by their GI (Glycaemic Index).

'The Glycaemic Index is a scoring system to show how quickly something gives up its sugars' says Ian. 'Ultimately, to avoid blood sugar spikes we want the foods we eat to give up their sugars slowly, which means we receive the resulting energy evenly over a period of time. The scale is open to interpretation but I think of something scoring over 100 as having a high GI, something medium would be between 35 and 60, and a low GI food would be something that scores under 35.

'A slice of white bread, for example, scores 100.

'While the Glycaemic Index is useful, it only tallies up items individually and, of course, we rarely eat foods in isolation. If you are measuring a combination of foods it's called a "glycaemic load". Here's an example. Let's say you have your piece of white bread which scores 100 on the chart, and you add jam to it. The jam scores 120, so you have 120 plus the bread, 100, totalling 220. Dividing this by two (as it's comprised of two elements, the jam and the bread) gives you 110, which is still a really high glycaemic score. But how about if you have the piece of bread with peanut butter on it? Peanut butter has a very low GI, say 30. So you have 30 and you have your white bread which is 100, add them together and divide them by two, it's 65. Now while that's still high, it's not as bad. It's worth being aware that measuring a product's GI is not a measure of health alone. Ice cream, for example, always scores low on the GI charts because it has lots of fat in it. Just looking at the Glycaemic Index alone is like looking at the calorie content of food without looking at the other nutritional information.'

'The masquerading sugars' (as Ian calls them)

These include honey and agave. While these items are often less processed than sugar, they are still used by the body in very similar ways. At about 60 calories per tablespoon, agave contains more calories per gram than table sugar, which has 40.

'The idea is this, just because something is "better" than something else, doesn't mean it's "good",' he says. 'Loading honey and agave onto a bowl of porridge isn't much better than loading it up with sugar. Often the difference is in the language used and the visual image it creates. When you think of honey you think of nature, bees, a nice sunny day, sunflowers, a lovely farmer in the countryside... When you think of sugar you think of plantations, factories, processing, the churning out of white granules, etc. But ultimately, from a nutritional standpoint, both are forms of sugar. We are not being duped by anyone, the public want to believe this [that some forms are better than others].'

STEP 2. KEEP A FOOD DIARY

Now you know what constitutes sugar and what does not, it's easy for you to keep a food diary. While I didn't do this on paper, I did evaluate all of my food choices to see if I was really getting a varied and balanced diet. The answer, as you know, was that I was not.

Keeping a food diary has really helped several of my more moderate friends who were on the fence about whether or not they ate a high-sugar diet. Recently, a group of four of them wrote down everything they ate and drank over a week as a challenge and the results really surprised them.

Sugar sneaks in to many things we eat and drink. A small packet of 'virtuous' sweet popcorn to see you through the afternoon: low in calories and fat, but sugar? Not so much. That 'odd' glass of wine you allow yourself actually adds up to about ten glasses by the end of the week.

Not only does it give you motivation to lower your intake once you have seen how much you are eating, keeping a food diary like this really allows you to see where easy low-sugar swaps can be made.

STEP 3. DECIDE WHETHER TO GO COLD TURKEY OR QUIT GRADUALLY

So, we now recognise sugar in all its forms and we have no excuses, but here comes the hard part. Giving it up. Advice varies on whether to go cold turkey or to cut down gradually. As you well know, I went cold turkey. Was this the easiest way? According to Ian, probably not. It was, however, the only way I could realistically do it.

I've already explained that it would be impossible to be 100 per cent sugar-free. Dairy has sugar in it, vegetables have sugar in them. Sugars occur, to some extent, in almost everything we eat. This means that cutting back on sugar can only be done in degrees.

I'm quite strict on myself for the vast majority of the time because I find it easier to avoid sugar completely than have a bit here or there. I also know I'm better at reacting to a dramatic change than the drip-drip effect of sticking to a small one. In other words, I favour the short, sharp shock method – getting it over quickly. It's so easy to procrastinate and delay the inevitable hard part for so long that I just end up losing momentum and slipping back into my old habits.

The good news is that Ian says going cold turkey doesn't have to be as hard as I made it. I probably hadn't adequately prepared my body for the shock of just giving up overnight, and as such I felt rather peculiar. But, there are supplements you can take (for recommendations, check my website www.sweetnothingbook.com) to support your system through the changes it will experience, which should ease any feelings of withdrawal. In other words, it doesn't need to be as horrid for you as it was for me. I'll let him explain.

'I wouldn't suggest someone cuts down their sugars overnight,' he says. 'They should plan it for a few weeks before. Begin by upping your magnesium levels either through your diet [so by eating more seeds, spinach, pulses and beans and quinoa] or by taking a supplement. Get into the habit of eating more lean protein that will help the body process sugar and curb cravings. I often suggest people start taking a good-quality probiotic to supplement their diet and keep their gut healthy, which also helps counteract sugar cravings.

'Start cutting back on your alcohol intake too. If you are going to lessen your sugar intake, alcohol is a good place to start. It has no nutritional value and provides lots of empty calories. The effects of it don't only last the day you drink a lot either. The day after you've overindulged on alcohol, your body craves a carbohydrate fix for both quick energy and to process the sugar already in your system. Drinking is a bit of a sugar-trap from that perspective.'

While I really advocate that people ditch sugar to as big an extent as they possibly can, I am all for people simply moderating their intake of sugar if that's all they feel they can realistically manage in their life. If this is you, go for it.

A lot of my friends – especially those with children – have decided to simply cut back on added sugar slowly, where they can. Their method is to gradually make healthier choices, but accept that from time to time they may err. All of them still eat fruit, lots of them still drink wine – 'but only at the weekend'. Unequivocally they have given up fizzy drinks, processed food and refined sugars. Here are some other really simple suggestions that can help you cut back on sugar:

◆ Swap your lunchtime sandwich or baked potato for a soup or salad with an olive oil dressing.

◆ Give up going to chain coffee bars. Not only are many of their coffee-type drink products choc-full of sugar, syrup and whatever else, their snack counters are stuffed with sugary cakes, biscuits and the like. Don't put yourself in the way of temptation. Save your money and buy yourself a new dress at the end of the month.

- ◆ Rather than buying a fresh juice on the way to work in the morning, get a cup of herbal tea or a water.
- ◆ Instead of reaching for a chocolate bar in the afternoon, have a handful of nuts or some vegetable crudités with hummus or tzatziki.
- ◆ Up your consumption of good fats by including full-fat plain yogurt with some toasted almonds and cinnamon in your routine, either as a pudding or a breakfast.
- ◆ Fall in love with avocados.
- ◆ Replace white rice with brown rice – it has a lower GI and reduces blood sugar spikes.
- ◆ Clear out your store cupboards and don't buy sweet food for the house. No biscuits, no crisps, no cakes, no fizzy drinks or cordial or other rubbish. If it's not there, you can't eat it.
- ◆ Don't drink alcohol. If you're going out and feel you need something, have a single shot of vodka, a squeeze of fresh lime, topped up with soda water. This is not only very low in sugar and calories, the soda water is rehydrating and counters the effects of the vodka.
- ◆ Throw away anything that has been artificially sweetened and any diet products that use low-calorie 'fake' sugars. I will explain why in Step 4.

STEP 4. REMEMBER THAT ARTIFICIAL SWEETENERS ARE NOT YOUR FRIEND

Think you can give up sugar and just get your sweet fix from a low-calorie alternative? Think again. Ditch that Diet Coke because research suggests that sweeteners – some of which are reported to be up to 13,000 times sweeter than sugar – may warp the body's perception of sweetness, causing us to overindulge. There has been much written about the negative effects of sweeteners on the body, including rumoured links to cancer and other horrible diseases. It must be stressed that no research has ever proven a link between sweeteners and cancer. However, recent research has shown that even drinking one artificially sweetened drink per day raises the risk of obesity, type 2 diabetes and metabolic syndrome as well as cardiovascular diseases. Long-term studies have also shown that consuming these instead of sugar doesn't necessarily help people lose weight.

Don't want to take my word for it? I don't blame you. After all, I'm not a scientist or even a nutritionist. But I think the clever folks at the Harvard School of Public Health in America know what they're talking about. I'm quoting the following from their website:

'One study of 3,682 individuals examined the long-term relationship between consuming artificially sweetened drinks and weight. The participants were followed for 7–8 years and their weights were monitored. After adjusting for common factors that contribute to weight gain such as dieting, exercising change, or diabetes status, the study showed that those who drank artificially sweetened drinks had a 47 per cent higher increase in BMI than those who did not.

'One concern about artificial sweeteners is that they affect the body's ability to gauge how many calories are being consumed. Some studies show that sugar and artificial sweeteners affect the brain in different ways.

'The human brain responds to sweetness with signals to eat more. By providing a sweet taste without any calories, however, artificial sweeteners cause us to crave more sweet foods and drinks, which can add up to excess calories.

'At the University of California in San Diego, researchers performed functional MRI scans as volunteers took small sips of water sweetened with sugar or sucralose. Sugar activated regions of the brain involved in food reward, while sucralose didn't. It is possible, the authors say, that sucralose "may not fully satisfy a desire for natural caloric sweet ingestion." So, while sugar signals a positive feeling of reward, artificial sweeteners may not be an effective way to manage a craving for sweets.'

In other words, when the body wants sugar, it isn't satisfied by us making do with an artificially sweetened product instead. It still wants 'real' sugar, and unless we have an iron will, we'll probably eventually give in and have some.

As simply stopping having sweetened products in the first place could eliminate this whole cycle, it's really worth doing so.

I'll let you into a little secret. Both I and my bezzy friend Jane used to be big fans of Diet Coke. I quit about three years ago after reading a lot of the negative publicity surrounding it, but before that, I got through two cans a day. Jane, however, works from home and was on another level. When I quizzed her about why she quit the habit at the start of 2014, she had a confession to make.

> 'I could get through six to eight cans of it a day. It's a dubious honour, but I could probably finish a can in about three mouthfuls. But I noticed that about 15 minutes after I'd finished one I'd want another and, as I'd always have an eight pack of it at home, I normally had one.'

As part of a general 'get-healthy' drive, Jane decided to ditch her habit, switching instead to water.

> 'I'm not sure if it is possible to be "addicted" to Diet Coke,' says Jane. 'I know Coca-Cola say it isn't. All

I know is that I really missed it when I quit. Water seemed boring, and when I went into the shop I would look longingly over at the cans. I can't deny that I would think about it throughout the day and miss not drinking it, but after two or three weeks of being strong, it stopped occupying my mind so much. It started me thinking, were someone to ask me to describe how Diet Coke tastes, I wouldn't know what to say. So I had a can the other week. I couldn't believe how horrible it was. Metallic, watery and just nasty. I suppose my palette has changed, but I can't believe I used to think it tasted good.'

Another interesting thing that Jane noticed is her evening sugar cravings have disappeared since ditching her Diet Coke habit.

'I haven't got what people would call a "sweet tooth",' she says. 'I'm not really into cakes or pudding, but for the past few years I've always rounded my evening off with a bar of chocolate. Since quitting diet drinks, I haven't felt a desire to do that. Perhaps this is for some other reason, but if so, after what you've told me about the Harvard information, it's an interesting coincidence.'

If you are really desperate to be able to add something to your tea, Ian Marber advises trying out Stevia, a natural herbal sweetener that's 200 times sweeter than sugar.

'The only sugar-substitute that is really worthwhile at the moment is Stevia,' he says. 'But Stevia has a slightly metallic taste, some say it tastes sort-of chemically. However, it's better than some of the alternatives.'

Not eating artificial sweeteners, by the way, extends to chewing gum and sugar-free mints. Some people credit both of these things with helping them to fend off sugar cravings, yet lots of gastroenterologists believe that the body starts expecting food when we chew gum, meaning it begins a digestive process, releasing more saliva, gastric and pancreatic fluids to help break down the expected food. Yet, of course as it's gum, nothing ever comes, which can upset the digestive system. Chewing gum is also thought to cause people to take down excessive amounts of air, which leads to stomach cramps, bloating and gas. Not good, people.

STEP 5. RE-PROGRAMME YOUR BRAIN

Are you an emotional eater? If you're someone who thinks of food as 'a reward', 'a treat', comforting or somehow a little bit 'naughty' then probably you are. That is to say you attach a meaning to eating which it doesn't need. Changing how you think about food will really help you stick to a healthier lifestyle.

I've spoken in depth about how I used to 'treat' myself on a daily basis – sometimes twice or thrice a day – for working hard. Or for getting things done, getting through the day. You know what I'm talking about.

To go low sugar, I had to totally transform the way I saw reward. Instead of bingeing on sugar, which is a very short-term fix, my reward these days is not eating the sweet thing, losing weight, looking better and feeling more healthy. I found it a simple choice, because unfortunately it's becoming increasingly plain that we can't have a high-sugar diet and look and feel well.

As Lee at Bodyism says:

'Before you start any life change, you need to work out what it is that really makes you feel good and what it is that you want to achieve. Then, ask yourself, will eating chocolate or whatever it is, help you achieve that?'

That's not to say you shouldn't enjoy food and see both cooking and eating as a huge pleasure. Food is more than just fuel for our bodies, it's a form of social bonding, a way of relaxing, nesting, showing someone you care.

'Going completely sugar-free is not only damn near impossible, but in absolutely simple practical lifestyle terms, making a food completely off-limits means you emotionalise your eating,' says Ian Marber. 'It means the same food – let's use chocolate as an example – can be seen by the same person as a "treat" one week, and a "punishment" the next, which it isn't, it's just a bar of chocolate.

When you really sit down and think about it, sugar is a strange thing to reward yourself with. It provides a momentary feeling, which actually gives you very little pleasure. It's fleeting, orgasmic; you enjoy it and then it's gone. Yet, the benefits of working hard and rewarding yourself by purchasing something you wouldn't normally buy – or an experience you wouldn't usually have – is obvious. In my book, that's more of a true reward.

But if you make food too much of a 'fuel' you take away all of the enjoyment. We just need to be grown up about it. We are grown up about all sorts of other things; if we are tired we go to bed early or we don't go out five nights a week, if our hair is dry we won't colour it five times in a month. We understand the consequences of doing silly things elsewhere in our lives, but when it comes to food we can often behave like children.

It's similar with drinking. Is that bottle of wine or

those four cocktails really going to be a long-lasting reward for you? Or is waking up without a hangover and feeling well your reward?'

Yet the great thing I found about giving up many forms of sugar is that after the first few weeks, I mostly didn't feel deprived – and nor will you.

Because they're no longer being bombarded by a plethora of incredibly sweet things, our taste buds adjust. Things that I didn't used to think tasted sweet, now do. Milk is the first example that pops into my head. Milk – which obviously contains lactose, a natural sugar – now tastes sweet to me. I've actually slightly gone off sweet potatoes as they taste too sweet, as do some varieties of squash.

But I am being completely honest in this book, so I'm not going to sit here and say I never miss sweet things or I don't sometimes really want to drink eight piña coladas back to back, just for a laugh. Of course, sometimes I do, as a one-off. The difference is, I wouldn't do it (and I haven't felt the need to do it) every day or every week anymore. Since I gave up most sugars two years ago, I haven't eaten one bag of Haribo or one bar of chocolate. In the interest of transparency – and for fear of one of the photographs being submitted to the press and my being exposed – I have eaten about six Bendicks Bittermints which my parents put in my Christmas stocking last year. They were my favourite. They were, of course, divine.

STEP 6. BUDDY UP

Do you know someone who also wants to ditch sugar? A workmate, your partner, your son or daughter, your teammate, a next door neighbour, a gym buddy? This challenge is much easier if you have a buddy to do it with.

If not, you can still do it. I did. But find yourself a mentor, whether that's me or someone else – there's also lots of support available online for when the going gets tough. I've already discussed how useful I found James Duigan's *Clean and Lean* books. They're available now as e-books, so you can take them with you wherever you go, which is helpful, but there are lots of other blogs and online low-sugar communities who share tips, tricks and recipes. Find and bookmark some of your favourites. Here are a few of mine:

◆ **www.sweetnothingbook.com** – This is my website. If you want help, support or just suggestions, come and find me here.

◆ **www.cleanandlean.com** – This is the original website from James and Christiane Duigan, featuring recipes, a shop and exercise suggestions.

◆ **www.deliciouslyella.com** – Ella is a young woman from London who was left almost completely bed-bound after being diagnosed with a rare heart condition. The self-confessed 'former sugar monster' decided to try and cure herself through food and it worked. Her nutritious low-sugar vegan recipes are, as the name suggests, completely delicious. Some of her recipes are more low-sugar friendly than others; go for the ones which don't use agave, maple syrup, honey and the like.

◆ **www.hemsleyandhemsley.com** – London-based sisters, Jasmine and Melissa Hemsley, make organic nutritious food, free from refined sugars, to keep you lovely, glowing and healthy, just like them.

◆ **www.goop.com** – Yes, it's Gwyneth Paltrow's website. I'm a big fan of her cookbook *It's All Good*, which was recommended to me by my friend Maya. The website is another great one-stop shop for healthy recipes.

STEP 7. REMOVE TEMPTATION

Earlier on in the book I talk about clearing out your cupboards. I can't over emphasise how important it is to do this. In the beginning, you will be very tempted. Perhaps you will buckle and have something contraband (I did with that cordial, remember?) – it's not the end of the world. But what will significantly reduce the chances of this is a good-old cupboard cleanse.

Throw away your sauces and jams, your meat marinades and all that delicious ice cream that's nestling in the back of your freezer. Frozen yoghurt can go too; it may be low fat, but take a look at yours (or ask, if you have a tendency to duck into an ice-cream parlour on a summer's day). It's almost certainly not sugar free.

Remember, fat doesn't make you fat.

Also, bin those processed foods. Don't eat your way to the end of the packet of biscuits or just make a deal with yourself to get to the end of this box of sweet cereal and not buy another. Get rid of it today. Put the bag outside in the wheelie bin and get excited about starting your new life.

Of course, if the desire is really that strong, you can go to the shop and buy something. We can all do that. It just takes a little bit longer – and a bit more effort. The aim here is to make it as difficult as possible to revert back to your old ways of eating – because they made you unhappy.

STEP 8. REPLENISH YOUR CUPBOARDS

Beauty editors are famous for their hero products, so I thought I could bring a touch of that glamour to your larder. I'm not including the obvious things here: vegetables, salad leaves, lean organic meats. But here are a few of my food hero products. Get them in and keep them in your store cupboard:

Coconut oil
Naturally cholesterol-free, coconut oil is heart-healthy, and although it's naturally sugar-free, it tastes sweet. It's also arguably the best oil for frying things as it's slower to oxidise so it's less damaged and chemically altered by heat during

frying. Some research has even shown coconut oil can help you lose weight. Best of all, it tastes divine.

It's not cheap but a little goes a very long way. Buy the solid, raw stuff that comes in a jar and not only can you cook with it, but you can eat it raw, add it to shakes, put a dollop in your porridge while you cook it on the hob (I never microwave food as it kills all the nutrients inside) and even use it on your hair or skin. You can get this pretty much everywhere now – Holland & Barrett, Amazon, independent health-food shops. I even saw it in Tesco recently.

Nut and seed butters

Whether you go for a no-added-sugar peanut butter, such as Whole Earth's crunchy one; almond butter, which is a bit more virtuous; or a seed butter, which is the most virtuous yet, nut and seed butters are a good way of getting your fats. Spread onto a couple of oatcakes, these make a good breakfast or snack.

Rolled oats, millet flakes, buckwheat groats, quinoa flakes

Experiment with these alternatives to wheat to create either a porridge-type mixture or a high-protein pancake batter recipe (see the recipe on page 188).

Full-fat organic yoghurt

No more low-fat for your body.

Alternative milks

Have you ever tried almond milk? Added to porridge or protein shakes, alternative milks are a great way to consume less dairy. Make sure you get the unsweetened versions or make your own. I've been making a wickedly tasty cashew nut milk with cinnamon lately.

Vegan protein powder

Let's get one thing straight: a little scoop of high-quality protein powder after exercising will not bulk you up and it won't make you look like a body builder. On the contrary. As and when you are ready to start exercising, a high-quality protein powder helps the body repair itself after a workout and it also helps create lean muscle, which is exactly what the new slimline you is after, right? I have tried a lot of different brands and my favourite is the Bodyism Protein Excellence Vanilla: no added sugar, low GI and vegan. At £50 for 500 g, this powder is an investment. However, you'll use it sparingly and it will last you months and months. It is available from the Bodyism website and Space NK stores or online.

Nuts

Whether you eat them as a snack or add them to recipes, prepare to fall back in love with the humble nut. High in protein and good fats, nuts are great for curbing cravings and regulating blood glucose levels, as well as being unbelievably healthy... in small doses. Because remember, as well as being tasty, nuts can be highly calorific, so try not to indulge in more than a handful. Macadamia nuts in particular are quite high in fat. When I say nuts, this obviously means plain nuts, not those covered in salt, batter, chilli flakes or dry-roasted flavourings. Sorry about that. If you can, try to buy the raw ones as their nutrients haven't been reduced by the heating process.

Avocados

Have half as a snack on oatcakes or at breakfast time to set you up for the day. I know it seems like a hassle. Those 'perfectly ripe' ones never really are, then you have to cut them in half and they're slippery little suckers. Getting the stone out = hassle; chopping it up and putting it in food wrap to try and ensure it doesn't go brown, again = hassle. But getting thinner? Having amazing hair, nails and skin? Feeling healthy and full of energy? So.Not.A.Hassle. Stock up on these babies now.

Smoked salmon

Yes, this lean protein is expensive, but you only need a couple of strips of it to really jazz up a meal. Scrambled eggs or smoked salmon and scrambled eggs. See what I mean? Go for organic so it's not too bright pink.

Eggs

These portable little babies are often deemed nature's 'perfect food' as they provide highly available protein as well as all the essential and non-essential amino acids, not to mention vitamins A, E and K as well as some of the B vitamins. Go organic and free range, research has shown that free-range eggs contain up to 20 times more omega-3 than eggs from caged hens.

Pumpernickel

This bread is low in fat, low in cholesterol, wheat-free and high in fibre. If you are missing bread made from wheat, this heavy, dark loaf made from rye flour may just do the trick. This isn't something to eat every day, but covered in mashed avocado for a weekend breakfast, it's hard to beat.

Dark green vegetables

These help to replenish the body's vitamins and minerals at times of stress.

Turkey

This meat contains an amino acid called L-tryptophan, which is needed to produce the body's calming feel-good hormone serotonin.

Feta or goats' cheese

Add interest to salads or frittata with these cheeses.

Mackerel

The *Clean and Lean Diet* book has a wonderful recipe for mackerel kedgeree made with brown rice, but I also like it for breakfast (although I have Scandinavian tastes!) and flaked into a salad with spinach, peas, cucumber and other bits and bobs.

Hummus

An ideal snack, rich in protein and fat, this garlicky chickpea dip is filling and nutritious.

Kale

It's a bit of a wonderfood is kale and, after enjoying a renaissance over the past few years, you'll find it available everywhere from farmers' markets to corner shops to huge superstores. This bitter, leafy green is surprisingly versatile. I like to add it to shakes, mix it with quinoa, topped with a poached egg at breakfast or bake it in the oven to make kale chips – a lovely crispy snack.

Seeds

Pep up a salad, perk up a soup or simply snack on these little protein-rich sources of joy. Toast them in the oven covered in herbs or spices to add a little more interest.

Chickpeas

While they have all manner of uses, including making your own hummus, I like to use chickpeas to stuff a free-range organic roast chicken. As the meat cooks, the flavours drip through the bird and into the stuffing mixture. It eliminates the need for roast potatoes. Indeed, Gordon Ramsay has a great recipe for roast chicken stuffed with spicy chilli chickpeas that you can find online.

Herbal tea bags

Find a brand that you enjoy – I love the Pukka brand as I think they taste best – and stock up. Brew up whenever you'd normally get a milky coffee.

Brown rice

With its extra bite and its more solid, robust consistency, brown rice takes some getting used to. It also needs a little more planning than cooking with white rice, as some varieties can take up to 40 minutes to cook. Don't let that put you off though. Rich in fibre and low GI, brown rice instead of white can make a big difference to your waistline.

Flavoured olive oils

My kitchen cupboard is home to a wide variety of different flavoured olive oils, from a peppery plain olive oil to a rich buttery one, and ones infused with fresh potent chillies, garlic or basil leaves. Get the best quality ones you can afford and keep and eat them at room temperature. These will become your marinades, your salad dressings and can be used in your cooking in lieu of other sauces and marinades which may contain added sugar.

Cinnamon

Some research has shown that as little as half a teaspoon of cinnamon every day can help reduce blood sugar levels, lower insulin resistance and curb cravings for sweet stuff. Aside from these great anti-sugar benefits, the warming spice also has a host of other benefits: it's thought to ease menstrual cramps, relieve congestion and help digestion. Plus, it tastes great either stirred into a cup of coffee with cream, or sprinkled over full-fat yoghurt or porridge. I can't get enough of this stuff.

Rather than focusing on what you can't eat on a low-sugar plan, it's good to look at what you can eat.

'As the body converts carbohydrates to sugar very easily,' Ian Marber says, 'it's fair to think of a low-sugar diet as effectively being a high-(lean) protein, high-(good) fat and low-carbohydrate diet.'

STEP 9. CHECK THE INGREDIENTS

As ingredients are listed by quantity, nutritionists normally agree that it's a bad idea to eat anything where sugar (and remember, sugar goes by several different names) appears in the first three ingredients listed.

It's a fairly safe bet that anything ending in –ose is a sugar. These have all been mentioned earlier in the book, but remember to pay special attention to added fructose, which goes straight to the liver. Anything that has syrup in the title, cane juice, molasses, dextrin, fruit juice pulp, fruit juice concentrate is also a secret sugar.

As you already know, sugar is also present in things that don't necessarily taste sweet. Sauces, canned salmon, certain varieties of fish fingers, some stock cubes. The list is almost inexhaustible.

Just because something is billed as healthy, or has implied health claims – 'low-fat', 'fat-free', 'contains no artificial ingredients' (you know the labels) doesn't make it free from sugar either.

Robert Lustig, author of *Fat Chance: The Bitter Truth About Sugar* has this to say on the subject:

> 'The Food Industry has contaminated the food supply with added sugar to sell more products and increase profits. Of the 600,000 food items in American grocery stores, 80 per cent have been spiked with added sugar; and the industry uses 56 other names for sugar on the

labels. They know that when they add sugar, you buy more. And because you don't know you're buying it, you buy even more.'

Don't be tricked into thinking that just because something sounds 'good for you', that it is. As Ian Marber says:

'Just because something is for example, organic, doesn't mean it's good for you. You can have organic pizza, organic chocolate... But your insulin is cold-hearted and brutal. It doesn't care that no pesticides have been used in the making of this. If there is sugar added to it or if it is something that's high GI, your body will react in exactly the same way whether it's organic or not.'

STEP 10. DEAL WITH THE CRAVINGS

Whatever it is that triggers our craving – a memory, stress, a bad day, seeing someone else eating something or simply habit – it's important to remember that you can head it off. Both time, and eating the right foods, will help you to beat your cravings.

Nutritional therapist Ian Marber believes that after the withdrawal phase, most cravings mean that something has gone wrong with our diets earlier in the day.

'Basically cravings often mean you have upset your body's glucose levels,' he says. 'Keep them balanced and you'll get significantly less cravings.'

Lee Mullins sees a lot of clients at the Bodyism gym who are starting out on a journey to give up sugar. I asked him how he helps people deal with the sugar demon on their shoulder.

'If people are craving sweets, you need to go back a step,' he says. 'Something wasn't right earlier in the day. Often it's sleep. If you're someone who doesn't sleep very well, then starts the day with a sugary breakfast to give you energy – often that's granola or toast and jam with a fruit juice, for example – you will be tired come 4 p.m. That's when you will "crave" something sweet like a chocolate bar, or something strong; perhaps a double cappuccino. There's no point addressing the craving itself, you have to fix the root cause of that craving in the first place. We often find that once people start sleeping better, they neurologically work better. Once that happens, they wake up with energy. If they're not feeling tired when they wake up, they make better choices for breakfast. All these things set you up for the day. If you sleep well and still suffer cravings, we would still advise people to look at their breakfast. No one should be starting the day with a large bowl of sugary cereal. Change that and you'll go a long way to countering your cravings later in the day. Helping someone sleep well and advising them how to choose a good breakfast changes their life.'

Nutritional therapist Ian Marber agrees.

'Once you have got past the beginning withdrawal stage of limiting your sugar intake, I would say most cravings mean that something has gone wrong earlier down the line. You have done something to unbalance your blood glucose levels – perhaps you've eaten too many quick-release carbohydrates for lunch. Basically cravings often mean you have upset your body's glucose levels. Keep them balanced and you'll get significantly less cravings.'

As well as watching what you eat for your main meals, try not to let yourself get too hungry. Carry a small packet of nuts in your bag, or a handy pack of oatcakes.

So, we know to up our intake of proteins and good fats, but is there anything else we can do? When I was going through some bad cravings, I asked Holly Pannett (as well as being my personal trainer she is also a qualified nutritionist) if there were certain foods that would help me quash cravings before they start.

'Cinnamon has been proven to help reduce cravings because it regulates blood sugar,' she said. 'Try adding it to your foods or your coffee whenever it goes. You do need to add quite a lot however – at least a teaspoon, which some people may find unpalatable, so I also tell people to take a great supplement from Lamberts Healthcare called Multi-guard Control. This multi-vitamin also contains magnesium, chromium and concentrated cinnamon. I advise my clients who are battling cravings to take two of these per day.

'Increasing the amount of chromium-rich foods you eat is another great way of controlling your blood sugar levels. Foods that are high in chromium include eggs, wholegrains, nuts, mushrooms, asparagus and liver and kidney, which may not be as palatable to modern tastes.

'Magnesium is also a bit of a wonder mineral. It's depleted by stress and if you're low you'll often find you feel more anxious, nervous or agitated. Eating a diet high in magnesium has been found to reduce chocolate cravings. If any of these things sound like you, try and eat more green leafy veggies; broccoli is an excellent source of magnesium as is spinach. Also

eat legumes (peas, beans, etc.) and wholegrains, such
as brown rice and figs.'

A handy tip for upping your magnesium levels came from
a friend and nutritionist, Anna King, who runs the London-
based Avocado Nutrition.

'One of the best ways to increase magnesium is Epsom
bath salts,' she says, 'as magnesium is well absorbed
transdermally [through the skin]. Add a cup to a warm
bath before bed and soak for 20 minutes. This is also
so relaxing and will help you drift off to sleep like
nothing else.'

STEP 11. KNOW HOW MUCH SUGAR IS ENOUGH

This is a difficult one. Even eminently qualified and experienced
nutritionists find it hard to set a blanket numerical target
on how much sugar people should eat – it's often down to
the individual, their lifestyle and their personal biochemical
make-up.

I've said this before at the start of the book but I think
it's worth repeating: the NHS says added sugars can safely
make up about 10 per cent of our daily calorie intake –
which means 50 g (12½ teaspoons) a day for women and

a whopping 70 g (that's 17½ teaspoons) per day, for men. While the NHS makes the usual disclaimers about the figures being dependent on people's age, size and levels of activity, many researchers claim these figures should be much lower or even halved to around six teaspoons a day for women and eight teaspoons for men.

Yet, in 2012, it was estimated, again by the NHS, that Britons currently eat a staggering 700 g of sugar each week on average. That's a whopping 175 teaspoons.

The interesting thing about these statistics is that, as a nation, we have fallen out of love with adding sugar to our foods. Sales of bags of sugar, so-called 'visible sugar' – i.e. the stuff we know that we're adding – have fallen. Yet we're still consuming more and more sugar because it is added to the majority of the ready-made foods we buy.

> 'It's standard advice that people shouldn't eat so much sugar,' says Ian. 'I keep my sugar intake low, I don't drink alcohol and rarely eat fruit. Every now and then I may buy a low GI fruit like blueberries. What's crucial about sugar is *how* you eat it, or in other words what you eat it with.'

So, if you are going to go low sugar rather than the whole hog, Ian advises combining your foods to limit the damage sugar does inside the body and avoid those blood sugar spikes.

'Avoid added sugar, and if you must have something that is naturally sweeter, only have it once a day with a balanced main meal – in other words something containing protein and fat to regulate your glucose levels. The sugar is more easily tolerated by the body this way. People like to look at foods in isolation, but it's a bit pointless because we don't eat foods in isolation. This is why sugary drinks are bad, they're packaged up with no protein and no fat and just go straight into your system. The disastrous combination is when you eat too much sugar with too much fat and too many carbohydrates.'

In other words, step away from the chocolate cake.

STEP 12. TAKE BABY STEPS

If it feels like too much of an ask for you to quit all sugars at once, do it gradually. Start by eliminating all added sugars – ready meals, processed foods like biscuits and cakes, muesli bars, fizzy drinks and anything you eat on the go. Simply eliminating these things will make a huge difference to your life and health.

Artificially sweetened low-sugar or sugar-free products that use man-made synthetic sweeteners should be ditched fairly early on, too. They make the body crave sweetness, which isn't what you want when it's the thing you are trying to cut back on.

Once you have conquered this, try to scale back your use of honey, agave and any other alternative sweeteners you have been using – apart from Stevia, the natural plant sweetener. If you sweeten your tea or coffee, start by reducing the quantities you add gradually until you are not having any. Replace sweetness on porridge and yoghurts with cinnamon, some dark berries and some nuts.

Once you have conquered those things, it's time to cut back on the high GI foods. Things like bread, pasta, white rice and the like haven't earned the right to be included in your new healthy regimen. They don't give you very much to help you through the day.

Lastly, gradually reduce your fruit intake. This process doesn't have to be drastic. You can do it over a period of weeks if you need to. The important thing is that you go back to seeing fruit as a delicious rarity rather than a 'healthy snack', there to be consumed at will. Replace your fruits with vegetables. Your body will thank you for it.

Chapter Six

LOW-SUGAR RECIPES

So now you know what you can't eat, it would be helpful for you to know what you can, right? I want you to know there is so much out there that you can eat. You won't feel deprived at all. As a general rule, most of the things you're making from scratch aren't going to have much sugar in them (obviously I'm not talking about baking). Fish, chicken or steaks served with veggies, salads, brown rice or other wholegrains are all going to be fine. Have fun, experiment, knock up some soups and big chunky salads full of good fresh things, using the best ingredients you can afford. There are lots of healthy food recipe books out there, so many that it's often hard to choose between them. As you know, in the beginning, I was desperate for inspiration, so I asked Holly Pannett, my personal trainer who is also a qualified nutritionist, to share with me some of her recipes and top tips for keeping food interesting yet healthy. While I often find myself short of time and cooking fish with brown rice and some veggies, all the following are also simple to make if you have company or want to spend a bit more time making something flavourful. We've picked the recipes that follow as some of Holly's true favourites – they're easy, tasty and 100 per cent good for you.

We've measured the ingredients in cups – it's a fairly universal way of measuring liquid and dry ingredients. You can get a cup measuring device (it often looks like a conventional measuring jug) from all cookshops, online stores and supermarkets.

BREAKFAST

Buckwheat and chia seed brekkie (serves 1)

Weekday breakfasts are something I really struggled with in the early days. Most of us simply do not have time to scramble eggs or make a healthy kedgeree before trundling off to work. This buckwheat and chia seed breakfast pot avoids all that morning stress. Simply make it the night before, drain it in the morning before mixing it together and you have a healthy nutritious breakfast that will have you good to go in no time.

¼ cup raw buckwheat groats (available from health-food
   shops)

2 tablespoons chia seeds

¾ cup unsweetened almond milk

small handful of raspberries or blueberries

¼ teaspoon ground cinnamon

The night before this is needed, soak the raw buckwheat groats in a bowl of water and leave overnight. This is done separately to the rest of the mixture as buckwheat groats take on a slimy texture when soaked.

In a separate bowl, whisk together the chia seeds, almond milk, berries and cinnamon. Whisk well until no chia clumps remain. Place in the fridge and leave overnight.

In the morning, put the buckwheat in a sieve and rinse thoroughly until no slimy pieces remain. Add the rinsed and strained buckwheat to the chia mixture and stir well.

Serve in a glass, topped with extra fresh berries if you wish.

Protein pancakes (serves 4)

This one is as easy as pie but you may have to play around with the ingredients to get the consistency right, depending on how thick or thin you like your pancakes. The good thing about this recipe is that it makes a big batch that will keep in the fridge for a few days. If you're making it for yourself and you whip it up on a Sunday, you've got a hearty supply of good-to-go breakfasts to see you through until Wednesday.

⅓ cup oats

1 cup cottage cheese

4 eggs

1 teaspoon coconut oil

2 teaspoons ground cinnamon

a dash of unsweetened almond milk

plain full-fat yoghurt, blueberries or toasted almonds, to serve (optional)

Put all the ingredients in a blender or food processor and whizz until it is a smooth batter. If the consistency is too thick, add a dash more almond milk. Once it's lump-free, transfer the mixture to an airtight container.

Heat a non-stick frying pan over a medium heat and spoon out a ladleful of your mixture into a frying pan. You shouldn't need to add any oil as the pancakes have oil in them and you're using a non-stick pan, but if you do, put a tiny amount of coconut oil into the pan just to grease it. You don't want the pancakes to fry. Cook until they are just starting to go brown and turn to do the same on the other side, then serve. I like these pancakes on their own, but you can add a dollop of plain full-fat yoghurt, a few blueberries, desiccated coconut or some flaked toasted almonds to serve.

Note: keeping the pancake batter in the fridge in an airtight container means you may have to add a touch more milk when you take the mixture out to use over the following days.

Coconut porridge (serves 1)

I love porridge; it's a filling and hearty way to start the day and like all the best weekday breakfasts, it's super simple. As with the pancakes, you may have to play around with the quantities here until you reach a consistency that you're happy with.

Coconut is one of the most nutritious foods known to man, containing vitamins, minerals and fibre, so the two combined make a heavenly combination!

½ cup oats

⅔ cup water

1 tablespoon ground flax or linseeds

6 tablespoons coconut milk

1 tablespoon coconut oil

toasted desiccated coconut or a few blueberries, to serve (optional)

Make this like you'd make any other type of porridge. Put the oats, water, ground flax or linseeds together in a saucepan with the coconut milk and warm over a low heat for about 6–8 minutes until it starts to bubble.

Take the pan off the heat, add the coconut oil and stir in.

Serve plain or with whatever topping you desire, whether that's some toasted desiccated coconut or some dark berries.

Pesto quinoa and kale breakfast bowl topped with poached eggs (serves 1)

Think you'll miss your big blow-out croissant and jam breakfasts at the weekend? Or that never-ending toast rack? Not with this recipe in your cooking arsenal you won't. Quinoa is a high-protein grain that comes dried and is incredibly easy to cook – simply boil as per the instructions on the pack. (In fact, I noticed in Sainsbury's the other day that you can buy ready-to-eat cooked vacuum-packed quinoa now. The packet I saw was by Merchant Gourmet, and it was next to the couscous.)

> 1 cup quinoa (any variety)
> 100 g shredded kale
> 2 eggs
> basil-infused olive oil
> ¼ avocado, chopped into chunks (optional)
> fresh pesto (optional)

Cook the quinoa according to the packet instructions.

Meanwhile, steam or boil the kale and set it to one side in a big bowl.

Put the eggs on to poach and set the timer for how you like them (4 minutes for soft, 6–8 minutes for hard boiled).

When your quinoa is cooked, combine it with the kale and stir in your avocado so it gets a bit warm and creamy, then drizzle with a little basil-infused olive oil. Transfer to a serving bowl and top with the poached eggs. A little dollop of fresh pesto can go on top, if liked. Mmm.

LUNCH

Broccoli and quinoa M & M (magnesium and manganese) super-salad (serves 4)

Magnesium and manganese help the body transport insulin

into the cell membranes and increase blood sugar levels. Low blood sugar levels often trigger cravings, so a diet rich in magnesium and manganese helps to control them. This recipe is both filling and tasty, the perfect recipe for a satisfying Saturday lunch.

1 cup quinoa

1 lemon

1 head of broccoli

1 tablespoon olive oil

6 anchovies

2 garlic cloves, crushed

¼ cup pumpkin seeds

salt and freshly ground black pepper

To cook the quinoa, simply add it to 2 cups of boiling water with the juice of the lemon and a pinch of salt. Leave it to cook for 15 minutes.

Meanwhile, chop the broccoli into bite-sized florets and set aside.

Heat the olive oil in a frying pan over a medium heat, add the anchovies and cook until softened and partially dissolved in the oil.

Add the crushed garlic and toss it around for a few seconds, taking the pan off the heat while you do this. You don't want the garlic to brown because it will then taste bitter and you want the anchovies to absorb the garlic flavour.

Add the steamed broccoli and toss this in the flavoured oil until it is well coated. The florets will soak up all the liquid.

Add the cooked quinoa and pumpkin seeds, season with salt and pepper and serve.

Grilled chicken and puy lentil salad (serves 4)

This high-protein salad works fantastically with grilled chicken, and leftovers can be taken to work for lunch the following day.

> 250 g ready-to-eat puy lentils (or you could soak green
>   lentils as per the instructions on the pack)
> 4 organic chicken breasts (optional)
> 2 tablespoons finely chopped or minced red onion
> a small bunch of chopped fresh coriander
> 2 tablespoons olive oil
> 150 g fresh mozzarella, diced
> 125 g thin-cut prosciutto slices, cut into strips

Heat the lentils for 4 minutes in a saucepan with 2 tablespoons of water. Put your chicken breasts, if you are using them, under a preheated grill to cook.

Meanwhile, mix the chopped red onion, coriander and olive oil in a serving dish, then spoon in the warmed lentils and gently mix.

Add the diced mozzarella to the mixture with the sliced prosciutto and serve.

Broccoli, cauliflower and leek soup (serves 5)

This soup is best served with a dollop of natural yoghurt and cracked black pepper.

> 2 leeks
>
> 1 tablespoon oil
>
> 1 head of broccoli
>
> 1 head of cauliflower
>
> 3 garlic cloves, crushed
>
> a 2.5 cm piece of fresh root ginger, peeled and sliced into matchstick-sized pieces
>
> 2 vegetable stock cubes

Wash the leeks, cut their ends off, quarter them lengthways, then slice into 1 cm pieces.

Heat the oil in a deep saucepan over a medium heat. Add the leeks and cook for 8 minutes until they soften but do not brown.

Meanwhile, cut the broccoli and cauliflower into florets and steam them until they are perfectly tender and a little soft. This will take 5–8 minutes.

Add the garlic and ginger to the pan of leeks and continue to cook for 3 minutes.

Dissolve the stock cubes in a jug containing 3 cups of boiling water.

When the broccoli and cauliflower are steamed, add the florets to a blender or food processor along with the leeks and one cup of the stock and pulse to blend. As you blend, slowly pour in the remaining stock until you reach your desired consistency.

SNACKS

Spiced crispy kale chips

Kale chips are enjoying what fashion people would call 'a moment' right now – Pret a Manger added them to their range at the start of the year and small brands such as Inspiral are bringing out their own flavoured ranges. Kale is a much hyped superfood and it's relatively inexpensive too. These are so easy to make and are great to have around when you've got the munchies.

> 1 head of curly kale or 1 bag of pre-chopped kale (use as much as your baking tray will allow. The kale needs to be spread across the tray in a single layer)
>
> 1 large tomato
>
> 3 sun-dried tomatoes
>
> 1 teaspoon olive oil
>
> 1 garlic clove, crushed
>
> ½ teaspoon paprika
>
> ½ teaspoon ground cumin
>
> sea salt and freshly ground black pepper

Preheat the oven to 180°C (350°F/Gas 4) and pop in a baking tray to warm up.

Wash and thoroughly dry the kale – any moisture will prevent the kale becoming crispy. Cut away and discard any stalks and place the kale in a large bowl. Bigger leaves work better for this as they don't go crispy too quickly. Try to ensure the leaves you have are of a similar size.

Put the tomato, sun-dried tomato, olive oil and crushed garlic in a blender or food processor and pulse to a smooth paste. Add the paprika, cumin, and some salt and black pepper and blend again until smooth.

Scrape the mixture into the bowl with the kale leaves. Toss the kale about to ensure the leaves are all evenly coated with a thin spread of the mixture. The intention is to add flavour, not cover the leaves with a thick coating.

Spread the coated leaves evenly over the warmed baking tray in a single layer and place the tray high in the oven. Leave the oven door slightly ajar and bake for 20 minutes until crisp, turning the leaves halfway through. Be sure to keep an eye on them, as different ovens will take slightly different times to cook. Do not let the leaves burn; they will crisp up as they cool.

Oomph orbs

(makes 12–15 depending on how big you make them)

These are great as a snack after a workout or if you are feeling low in energy. They're quite calorific, so one a day is adequate. Because this recipe makes quite a few, you can afford to be generous and give them to your friends!

½ cup nuts (a mix of almonds, brazil and walnuts or just
almonds on their own)

½ cup dried figs (the squishier ones work best)

1 teaspoon melted coconut oil (this is just so the mixture
does not stick to your hands)

1 teaspoon vanilla essence

2 tablespoons shelled hemp seeds

3 tablespoons desiccated coconut, to coat

Start by pulsing the nuts in a food processor until they are finely chopped.

Add the figs and blend again until the mixture comes together in a smooth paste. Add the melted coconut oil and vanilla essence and pulse again.

Scrape the mixture out onto a board and knead in the hemp seeds with your hands. Roll the mixture into small balls and coat with desiccated coconut or more hemp seeds if desired.

Place the orbs in the freezer to set for 20 minutes. These are best kept in the fridge in an airtight container. They should last for a few days.

Sweet potato protein slab (about 10 servings)

Nowadays it's quite common to use sweet potato in baking – a friend of mine makes brownies using sweet potato. But this protein slab is one of my favourite weekend treats and is ideal when you're on the go or after you return from the gym. It's more convenient than eating a chicken breast or trying to make a protein shake if you're not at home.

coconut oil

1 small sweet potato, peeled and cut into large chunks

2 scoops protein powder (I like Bodyism's Vanilla Protein Excellence but any whey protein isolate is ideal, either a vanilla or an unflavoured variety)

2 heaped tablespoons almond butter (drain any excess oil on a piece of kitchen towel)

1 tablespoon ground cinnamon

8 dried apricots, chopped

8 tablespoons buckwheat groats

Grease a small shallow baking dish with coconut oil.

Put the sweet potato in a saucepan of boiling water and cook for about 15 minutes, until soft. Drain and leave to cool, then place in a blender and blitz to make a rough puree.

Mix the protein powder, almond butter, cooked sweet potato and cinnamon together in a bowl. Add the chopped apricots and buckwheat groats and combine. Spoon the mixture onto the greased baking tray.

Place the tray in the freezer to set for 1 hour. Cut the slab into protein bar shapes. These should last 3–4 days.

DINNER

Super saag (serves 6 as a side dish)

Sometimes only a curry will do. I've already described how many takeaway meals are absurdly high in saturated fat, salt and other nasties, and the only true way to avoid this is to make your own. This super saag uses spinach to great effect – you'll be gently plenty of vits without even knowing it.

500 g fresh spinach leaves

1 tablespoon butter

6 garlic cloves, finely chopped

1 onion, finely chopped

½ a tomato, finely chopped

200 ml unsweetened almond milk

½ teaspoon salt

¼ teaspoon garam masala

¼ teaspoon ground coriander

¼ teaspoon ground cumin

¼ teaspoon turmeric

a small handful of chopped fresh coriander

Steam the spinach for 15 minutes, then pop it into a food processor and blend.

Heat the butter for 30 seconds in a frying pan over a medium heat, add the garlic and cook until it is soft. Add the onion and cook for a further 2 minutes. Add the blended spinach and tomato and the almond milk.

Add the salt, garam masala, ground coriander, ground cumin, and turmeric. Cook for a further 3 minutes over a high heat. Finish by adding the chopped fresh coriander before serving.

Tarka dahl-ing (serves 4)

This dish is lovely served with brown rice and a tangy raita (a yoghurt, cucumber and mint dip).

> 1 tablespoon olive oil
>
> 1 teaspoon mustard seeds
>
> 1 teaspoon cumin seeds
>
> 4 garlic cloves, finely chopped
>
> 2 fresh green chillies, deseeded and finely chopped
>
> 1 tomato, finely chopped
>
> 1 onion, chopped into small cubes
>
> 250 g lentils – green, red or yellow, soaked in water for at least 1 hour and drained (this makes them easier for the body to digest)
>
> 1 teaspoon salt
>
> 1 teaspoon turmeric
>
> 2 teaspoons ground coriander
>
> 1½ teaspoons ground cumin
>
> a handful of chopped fresh coriander

Heat the oil in a deep saucepan or even a wok over a high heat for 1 minute. Add the mustard and cumin seeds and heat for a further minute to release the flavours.

Add the garlic and green chillies to the warming seeds and reduce to a medium heat. When the garlic starts to go soft, add the finely chopped tomato and onion and fry for a further 2 minutes.

Add the soaked and drained lentils and 500 ml boiling water. Add the salt, turmeric, ground coriander and ground cumin.

Cover with a lid and cook the dahl for 12–15 minutes, stirring every 5 minutes.

Scatter the handful of chopped fresh coriander on top of the dahl before serving.

Grilled salmon with rocket, aubergine and red pepper salad (serves 4)

This dish is filled with different colours and textures – from the nutty bite of the pecans to the soft, melting texture of the salmon and aubergine, it's like a festival on a plate.

2 red peppers, deseeded and sliced

2 aubergines, sliced

3 tablespoons olive oil

2 large sweet potatoes

1 teaspoon paprika

4 salmon fillets

1 lemon

1 cup pine nuts

½ cup pecans

    1 teaspoon agave

    1 teaspoon ground cinnamon

    salt and freshly ground black pepper

    1 bag of rocket leaves, washed and dried

For the dressing:

    3 tablespoons olive oil

    juice of 2 limes

    ½ teaspoon sea salt

    ½ teaspoon black pepper

    2 tablespoons water

    2 teaspoons tahini

Preheat the oven to 180°C (350°F/Gas 4). Place the sliced red peppers and aubergine on a baking tray, drizzle with 2 tablespoons of the olive oil, and sprinkle with salt and pepper. Roast in the oven for 15 minutes, turning the veggies once halfway through.

Remove the skin from the sweet potatoes and discard. Continue to peel the potatoes so that you have long slivers. Place the slivers in a bowl with the paprika and the remaining olive oil, season with salt and pepper and mix.

Once the peppers and aubergines have roasted for 20 minutes, add the sweet potato slivers and cook for a further 12 minutes.

Preheat the grill to a high setting. Prepare the salmon fillets by placing them on a baking tray lined with foil. Season with salt and pepper and squeeze the juice of 1 lemon over the fillets. Place the tray under the grill and cook for 8–10 minutes.

Meanwhile, place the pine nuts and pecans in a frying pan over a low heat and gently toast them with the agave syrup and cinnamon for about 3 minutes.

As the hot ingredients cool, combine the ingredients for the dressing in a bowl. Arrange the rocket leaves on 4 serving dishes, stack the roast veggies on top, drizzle over the dressing and sprinkle over the toasted nuts. Finally place the grilled salmon fillets on top, then serve.

FOR A SPECIAL OCCASION

Black bean brownies (makes 16)

As a rule, I try to avoid desserts, but if you are making food for friends, sometimes only a pudding will do. These brownies are best served in smaller portions as they have a real chocolatey kick.

    3 tablespoons melted coconut oil, plus extra for greasing

    1 tin black beans (425 g)

    2 eggs

    ½ cup good-quality cocoa powder

    2 tablespoons ground cacao nibs

    ¼ teaspoon salt

    1 teaspoon vanilla essence

¼ cup agave

1 ½ teaspoons baking powder

2 tablespoons unsweetened almond milk

50 g 85 per cent cocoa solids dark chocolate, chopped

Preheat the oven to 160°C (325°F/Gas 3)and grease the holes of a mini-muffin tin with coconut oil.

Rinse and drain the black beans well. Combine the beans, eggs, coconut oil, cocoa powder, cacao nibs, salt, vanilla essence, agave and baking powder in a food processor or blender and blend for 3–4 minutes. You may need to add a tablespoon of almond milk to get the consistency right – you are aiming for a creamy velvet, but not runny batter. Mix in the chopped dark chocolate so that it is speckled throughout the mix.

Spoon the mixture into the muffin tins and place on the middle shelf to bake for 17 minutes. The finished brownies should remain soft and gooey in the middle. Kept in an airtight container, these should last for about three days.

Chocolate mousse – avocado style (serves 4-6)

We know that when we eat sugar it's best to accompany it with fat and protein as these things help keep your blood sugar levels stable. Combining cocoa, dates and banana with avocado is a good way to do this. You can substitute the dates and banana with 2 tablespoons of agave if you want. I prefer not to.

100 g 85 per cent cocoa solids dark chocolate

3 very ripe avocados (if you need to speed this process
up, try placing avocados in a brown paper bag with a
banana or tomato, or wrap them well in newspaper –
the trapped ethane gas will speed up the process)

¼ cup good-quality cocoa powder

1 ripe banana

4 medjool dates

2 tablespoons ground cocoa nibs

1 tablespoon vanilla essence

¼ teaspoon sea salt

fresh raspberries or chopped toasted hazelnuts, to garnish
(optional)

Break the dark chocolate into squares and melt slowly in a glass bowl set over a pan of simmering water – making sure the water does not touch the base of the bowl.

Peel and stone the avocados and place them in a bowl with the cocoa powder, ripe banana, medjool dates, cocoa nibs, vanilla, salt and melted chocolate and whisk for 4 minutes until a desired texture is reached.

Spoon the mixture into small ramekin dishes and garnish with fresh raspberries or chopped toasted hazelnuts. Leave the mousse in the fridge for 3 hours to set and serve immediately.

Chapter Seven

FITTING LOW SUGAR INTO YOUR LIFE

I'm two years in now, so you're probably thinking that I find being low sugar easy, right? Wrong.

While I do find it enjoyable, I don't find it easy. I was raised eating sweetened foods. By the time I stopped, I'd been living on my own, cooking and shopping for myself for over 15 years – and for all of that time, several times a day, I had been eating sweetened foods. Two years 'clean' is a drop in the ocean in the face of that.

Giving up is the easy bit. If you've ever been on a diet, decided to get fit or tried to give up smoking you'll know, it's not starting the change that's difficult, it's sticking to it.

But persevere and I am certain that, in a few weeks, you will find yourself enjoying your life more than you have in a long while. I know this, because it's what's happened to me.

I'm not an angel, but as many of my family members and former boyfriends can testify, I am incredibly stubborn. If I think I am right, I will debate something until everyone else gives up. I like to win arguments and I rarely let something beat me. I think my stubbornness is what's given me good willpower. Indeed, since I started this back in June 2012, I have always been determined not to allow my dependency on sugar to beat me. But, at times, I have felt sorely tested by my decision to be low sugar.

While I have never fallen off the wagon for any significant portion of time, there have been days when I've had a bit of a blow out.

A few months ago, for example, I'd had a hard few weeks. As a freelance writer, my work schedule is either feast or famine. After a while of not working very much, lots of projects came in and I had five deadlines in one week. On top of this, there was love stress. I'd been putting off some hard personal decisions I knew I had to make concerning a relationship – namely, whether I should invest any more effort into it, or just let it fizzle out. Harrumph. My brain felt busy, wired, overwhelmed with thoughts.

So, when Saturday came around – and with it a longstanding plan to see Katy and get our hair done before going out for drinks in glamorous Notting Hill – I knew my resolve would be tested. Katy and I were offered cocktails in the salon; she got a glass of champagne and, at first, I ordered a water. But as the appointment wore on, I mentioned my love of White Russian cocktails – a drink made from vodka, Kahlúa (an ultra-sweet coffee liqueur) and full-fat milk or cream, served over ice. The next thing I knew, I was ordering one 'just in case' I wanted it. Normally I resist temptation, but on this day, I just went for it. Dear reader, although it was only 3 p.m., I drank a White Russian – through a straw. It was strong. And heavenly.

But, of course, it was a slippery slope. About an hour later in lovely bar I had a glass of red wine – yes, bad combo – by which time I felt rather tipsy because I rarely drink these days. So, of course, I followed it up with a large bowl of chips and mayonnaise. Hmmm.

Don't get me wrong, I know that in the grand scheme of life, a cocktail, a glass of red wine and a big bowl of chips and dip isn't the end of the world. Most would say it was fairly moderate, and to be honest, I'd agree. But I could feel where this was going. It was descending into a period of what I call 'spiralling' – where things go further and further off course until they're totally out of control. It was very much the lifestyle of the old me. So that's when I decided I had to leave. I was home on the sofa by 8 p.m., feeling a bit wired.

Another situation that always tests my willpower is being at my parents' house in Sussex. Mum and Dad have lived in the same nice semi-detached house since I was two years old. It's the only family home I have ever known. Although my parents have long since consigned my Pearl Jam, Hole and Nirvana posters to the recycling bin and carpeted over my drafty, stripped floorboards, my bedroom is in all other respects the same. Much to my dad's fury, it still has two wardrobes full of cool vintage clothes that I used to wear as a teenager and the Laura Ashley 'Forget Me Not' bridesmaid's dress I wore at my cousin Alison's wedding when I was nine.

As a grungey 16-year-old I spray painted my wardrobe doors and scrawled the name of a band I was in – the rather aptly named 'Sugar Baby' – in black eyeliner pencil on the side of the closet. It's all still there.

Naturally then, sleeping in the same bed, being in the same room, it's very easy to want to slip back into the same eating habits. I find myself always looking longingly at the countertop where they keep the fizzy pop. My parents also have a biscuit tin that often comes out on a weekend afternoon around 3 p.m., or later in the evening while we're watching television. Of course, there will almost always be some form of chocolate somewhere, or a piece of buttered malt loaf or toasted teacakes or all of the above. There are jumbo bags of dry-roasted peanuts and plain nuts with dried fruit. A pudding option comes with every meal.

While my mum is probably one of the nicest, most caring people in the whole world, she does not understand the low-sugar thing, despite my explaining it several times. For example, pretty much every time I go home she offers me Frosties or granola for breakfast. Bless her, I love her, but if we're ever in her car together, she'll offer me a humbug or a Werther's Original from the glove box.

'I know you don't eat sugar, but do you want a piece of yule log?' has been the question asked of me, two Christmases running.

Me: 'No thanks, Mum, it's very sugary.'

Mum: 'Okay, how about a small bit of Christmas pud? It's a nice one, and it's really only fruit. Mostly... Or a mince pie? Have a mince pie.'

Me, looking at the icing sugar coated mince pie dish: 'No thanks, Mum.'

She frowns.

It's interesting that even after two years of being low sugar, I still sometimes find it hard, especially when I am out of my normal routine. Although I'm no longer swayed by a wine list or a pudding menu at a restaurant, the low-toned rattle of a box of Maltesers being passed between family members at my dad's birthday a few months ago sent me into a paroxysm of longing.

This is one of the many reasons I still feel that – despite what the experts say – sugar is addictive. While it doesn't cause such noticeable anti-social effects as dependencies on alcohol, tobacco or drugs – and, of course, I am not attempting to belittle those issues or affiliate a liking for a bar of Dairy Milk with injecting heroin – sugar is also incredibly hard to give up. Yes, the physical symptoms of withdrawal are debilitating but they are, at least, short term. As with other addictions, the emotional attachment lasts long after you've quit the habit. Worst of all, as sugar is socially acceptable, it's almost impossible to avoid.

'There is a link between consumption of carbohydrates and our perception of happiness, it's a dopamine connection. In other words, when you eat anything you like or enjoy, your brain will create dopamine,' says Ian Marber.

Getting a dopamine fix is one reason we miss sugar (which is of course a carbohydrate) so much when we give it up. So I asked Ian, does this mean if I were brought up to believe that kale was a treat, would I have the same response and feeling when I ate that as I used to get from eating a bag of pick-n-mix?

'Well, the body has a biochemical dopamine response when you eat carbohydrates – this can't be helped, but if you were brought up to believe that kale was in some way a "reward food" like other things, your brain would release a bit of dopamine when you ate it, yes.'

I asked Lee Mullins of Bodyism if everyone he sees finds it hard to stay off the white stuff.

'Cutting back on sugar in foods is the hardest life change for our clients,' he says. 'Sugar in drinks –

alcohol – is actually pretty easy to give up. On average, people drink alcohol about three times a week so when it comes down to it, most people can take it or leave it. But sugar in food is everywhere. It can creep in three times a day, every day, in some form or another. We're never going to say to someone who really wants it that a glass of good-quality red wine once a week is going to be harmful to them – in fact it has some health benefits. But it's probably not going to help them drop any fat if that's what they're trying to do, because it slows the whole process down. Having a glass of wine every night is not going to be great for you.

'This is because sugar [and a medium-dry wine can have about 0.5 to 2 g of sugar per glass] is an antinutrient. It actually depletes your body of nutrients. Without them, the body feels tired, it can't repair, it can't build and grow or stay youthful and young. Sugar makes your body age faster. No one wants that'.

This is where what I talked about in the last chapter really comes in to play. You have to change your life, create a new lifestyle that works with your new regime. Lee had some good advice on this.

'Lots of our clients have high-powered jobs,' says Lee. 'They need to wine and dine clients and to an extent drinking goes with the territory. We work with people to find ways around that, because going low-sugar really does involve a whole lifestyle change. So if someone's work involves a lot of client dinner meetings, we ask them if they can perhaps make those dinners breakfasts instead... It's frowned on to have whisky with your eggs at breakfast! Breakfasts and lunch meetings are safer than dinner meetings if you are trying to overhaul your lifestyle.

'If that's not so much you, but you have issues with going out with friends – say you experience quite a lot of peer pressure – try driving to a night out. Just small changes like that make a huge difference and help you stick to your new lifestyle.'

Personally speaking, a large part of changing my lifestyle was accepting the fact that although I had some healthy-looking slender friends who seemed to be able to turn up to work in the morning eating a pain au chocolat and drinking a large latte and never put on a pound, or didn't seem to feel super tired and irritable, that wasn't me. I am never going to be the girl who 'gets away with it'. An excessive sugar consumption doesn't agree with me – in fact it doesn't really agree with anyone. Its effects on me are just more evident.

Lee's not only a personal trainer who tells other people what to do, he's also experienced the negative side of sugar.

'I was a football player for years, so I've always been mindful of being healthy,' he says. 'I couldn't go out and drink then get up and play football the next day. Although I've never been a big drinker, I did sometimes have a few. But when I did, it just didn't work for me. I would wake up and feel so awful I'd stay in bed the whole day and I wouldn't do anything. Then, before I knew it, it was Monday and I was up and going to work again. I felt like I had no time to do anything, which was frustrating as I really cherished my time off.

'It didn't take long for me to realise that drink and I weren't very compatible. Of course at the beginning my friends didn't like it. I was a 17- or 18-year-old guy who didn't drink. But I changed the way I went out with my friends. Instead of going to the pub I'd meet them for lunch, go to play football, go to the gym. If I went out in the evening, I'd drive everywhere, which meant I couldn't drink. Basically I just didn't put myself in that position.'

But what if someone else puts you in that position? What if your neighbour buys you a box of Bendicks for Christmas because they're 'your favourite' (they are) and sits down with you to tuck in over a cup of tea, meaning you eat six in quick succession? Do you say 'Oh sorry, I don't eat these now,' and hand them back?

Or how about you and five other people go to a friend's house for dinner to find out she's made pulled pork – a dish that's been sitting marinating in sticky sugars before being slowly cooked with great care for hours on end – served in white bread buns with a sweet barbecue sauce and chips? Do you tell her you can't eat it and instead get out your emergency packet of oatcakes while everyone else is tucking in?

These are two true examples of things that have happened to me at the start of this year, and you know what, going low-sugar is pretty easy if you live on your own – as I do – or with someone else who's also happy to go along with you and make all these changes. When you have your larder stocked with walnut halves and chia seeds and a fridge with almond milk nestled inside the door, sticking to a regime like this is a breeze. But what about in other situations? Indeed, what I eat when I'm going out for dinner or around at someone else's house is the focus of the most commonly asked questions that get fired at me when people find out about my dietary habits. Here are the answers:

At a dinner party

When it comes to dining out at someone else's house, I normally just eat what I'm given. After this amount of time, most of my friends and acquaintances know I don't eat sugar and cater accordingly. If I'm invited over, however, I never remind them of it or ask what they're going to make. I don't want to be neurotic and controlling over other people's diets, and besides, as I've already discussed above, it's not the end of the world if what I'm given doesn't tally with what I'd normally eat. Embrace the change.

But, say I've been invited round by someone who I don't know well and they ask me if there's anything I don't eat... what to do then?

Well, I've made it a rule not to say this: 'yes actually, just sugar', the reason being that I know it will have them doing cartwheels of despair around their kitchen as soon as they've put the phone down. Instead I say, 'oh not really, but I don't have a massive sweet tooth so am not too keen on puddings' and leave it at that. It's about managing expectations. Most of the time, homemade foods that are cooked from scratch are actually pretty fine.

As well as taking a bottle of wine or flowers for the hosts, I always bring a bottle of fizzy water for myself. Sometimes, if I'm feeling generous or I know the hosts are big pudding eaters I take a selection of cheeses that I like (I know! Selfish!) with some oatcakes, which they can whip out at dessert time. This not only makes you seem ultra-generous, but it doesn't make you feel as if you're abstaining when everyone else is oohing and aahing over their gooey chocolate torte and you have nothing on your plate.

Travelling

Let's be honest, it's not easy to be low sugar if you are on the go. I mentioned my petrol station problem earlier in the book, but motorway services are by no means alone in almost exclusively providing junk food for journeymen and women to snack on. Take train stations, for example. The other day I took a train from London's Victoria Station. Krispy Kremes, cupcakes, sweets, pick-n-mix (another old favourite), sandwiches, Burger King, McDonald's, a sushi store, coffee chains… you get the picture. None of these places is ideal. In the end I found a Pret a Manger over the road and grabbed a bag of their tasty (and, at £1.50, pricey) kale chips, which I highly recommend. (Indeed Pret are quite good at providing small bags of tasty roasted nuts too, if you're ever caught on the hop. Steer clear of their green juices though, which have recently been revealed to be very high in sugar.)

By far the worst travel culprit are newsagents with their rows upon rows of chocolates, sweets, crisps, miniature cakes, fizzy drinks, biscuit bars and the like. In their defence, I am sure some probably sell plain nuts, but I tend to avoid shops like these. You can't even buy a newspaper in the morning without them trying to flog you a huge sugar-bomb bar of chocolate wrapped in pretty metallic paper for half its normal price.

Airports are not much better. I travel quite a lot for both work and fun, and have developed a little ritual that works for me. Whether you're going low sugar or not, it's never a wise idea to drink on a flight – I have learnt this the hard way. Most people know that one alcoholic drink in the air is the same as three on the ground and although I did once get rather tipsy aboard a flight to New York with a very handsome rock climber which was fun, you always feel terrible the minute you get to passport control.

Nowadays, mine's a spicy tomato juice if it's fresh, or a fizzy water if it isn't. I also take a couple of litres of water on the plane with me.

Then there's food. If I'm on a relatively short-haul flight (under seven hours), I don't eat the meal that's served. I know it sounds pretty boring and it leaves you with yet more time to fill in the air, but I try to buy something nice to eat at the airport before I get on the plane, then take something else – a salad, a wrap or whatever it may be – to pop open when the meal is coming around if I'm hungry. From time to time (depending on what class you're travelling in) you'll be pleasantly surprised that the meal actually is something you'll want to eat, but most of the time the food is a processed, salty, squidgy mess that isn't really worth the calories. This is certifiably, definitely always true of breakfast on a night flight. Some horrible sweaty muffin filled with bright pink goo, or an ultra-refrigerated fruit salad? Tough choice, but no thanks. Try to take as many snacks as your hand luggage will allow – I always take oatcakes (again, I know) and whatever else I can fit in my bag that won't be confiscated by the security guys.

If you've forgotten or can't be bothered to carry lots of stuff, most airport terminals now have a Marks and Spencer Simply Food where you can buy either little carrot and celery batons with hummus or nice bags of nuts and wasabi peas, which are good for emergencies.

Around children

Not having children of my own, this is a hard one for me, but the matter is understandably so complex and lengthy it could be a book in its own right – and maybe it will be. Conventional packaged children's food is often loaded with sugar or sweeteners, which obviously isn't massively beneficial for kids or anyone looking after them. The only way around this is to make them the same food that you are making yourself and gradually wean them off whatever 'treats' they are being given by grandparents, etc. – bottled fruit juice drinks and the like. I think it's important not to be seen as having any food hang-ups around kids. I try to be quite careful around my nieces, Millie, six, and Matilda, one, after I heard Millie telling people that I don't eat much sugar 'because it's bad for you'. She'd obviously heard me explaining something to my mum or sister. While I may believe this to be true, I'm not sure putting my opinions about food onto a child is a wise idea so now I try to reign in my comments on food around them.

On holidays

This is a hard one for lots of people. Again, it depends where you go. Florida, land of fresh orange juice and big breakfasts = hard. New York, city of gym-goers and vegan, gluten-free, low GI, organic salad bowls = easy. The same goes for holidaying in the Mediterranean, where grilled fish, salads and rice are often the order of the day. Wherever I am, I try to always have oatcakes (I am not sponsored by Nairns, I promise!), nuts and any other snacks that I'm attached to at that precise moment because jet-lag often means you're hungry at strange times. Make sure you keep hydrated by drinking lots of water as this will stop you from wanting to snack so much. Then, just do the best you can – and enjoy yourself.

Lunches at work

Living in London or any big city tends to mean that there's a lot of choice when it comes to buying your lunch. Whether it's the canteen salad bar, a trip to a sandwich chain, a little independent place or a health-food eatery, there's not really much you can't lay your hands on within a very short radius of your office. But what happens if you are trying to follow this plan while living in rural Derbyshire or the Pennines?

Being honest, you should probably take your lunch in to work. The easiest way to do this is to make a bit extra of whatever it is you ate the night before. Lots of the recipes I know and love – from *Clean and Lean*'s mackerel kedgeree to Holly's tarka dahl-ing (see page 200) – taste just as good heated up the following day (obviously be careful when it comes to reheating rice). If your office has a microwave or a hob, cook it through until it's piping hot and then chow down. Soups are great and easy, huge salads too.

If you're wedded to your sandwiches, you can get amazing speciality breads now – spelt, rye, amaranth and the like – which means you can fill your sandwich void without eating highly processed white or brown bread, and as you know, there are always, *always*, oatcakes which you can top with smoked salmon, hummus, avocado, beetroot. Take a little pot of full-fat natural yoghurt with you if you feel you need to round off your meal with something that's not savoury.

Snacking

There are certain things I always have in my drawer at work. I'm not going to mention the first one, but it has eight letters, starts with an 'o' and ends with an 's'. The next is a jar of ground cinnamon. Whether it's to add to a cup of coffee, to top off a desk-based breakfast of porridge or to sprinkle onto a plain yoghurt, a jar of ground cinnamon is a good desk gonk to have to hand if you need a flavour hit but want to keep it natural. Nuts as well, of course.

If you're a person who likes crisps, go for some organic corn chips – you know the ones that are like Doritos, but without all the flavourings? Get plain if you can, lightly salted if you have to. I like the R. W. Garcia Organic Blue Corn and Flaxseed ones, which are available from lots of places and also on Amazon. These are great for dips if you're having people over, served with a good homemade guacamole, hummus or baba ghanoush (aubergine dip). Beware, however, these corn chips are pretty moreish.

While I talk about snacking a lot, try to ensure you're only eating when you are hungry and not just when you're bored or in need of something to do. This sounds really obvious I know, but when you think you are hungry, first have a glass of water – the body often misinterprets dehydration as hunger – and then see if you still feel hungry.

Dinners out

For me, this is the easiest time to be low sugar if you bear in mind a few key rules:

- Shy away from anything with a sauce. The more gloopy the sauce, the worse it is. Gravy, for instance, probably not too bad. A hoisin or a black bean sauce at a Chinese restaurant? Not so good.
- Always avoid the bread basket. If you are super hungry before you leave to go out, have a few nuts or

something at home to tide you over.

◈ Puddings are a no-no. Even when you go out. If you want to end the meal with something, have some cheese, but ideally try to go without.

◈ Wine – not if you can help it. Driving will help you avoid this issue, but if it's really a problem or you'd really like a glass, go for a nice glass of red wine alongside a big glass of water and sip it slowly while you eat. Wine is lower in sugar than many types of beer, so it's a better choice.

Certain cuisines are more low-sugar friendly than others:

◈ Going to a steak house, a French restaurant or a grill means there's pretty much always something you can eat – a grilled fillet steak with spinach or a salad, for example.

◈ The same goes for fish restaurants, so if I'm meeting someone out, I often try to book us in to one of these places.

◈ If you go to a burger place, ask them to keep the bun and go easy on the ketchup and mayonnaise.

◈ Going to an Asian restaurant starts to become a bit more problematic – stir-fries with little or no sauce are fine, but many Thai, Chinese, Indonesian and Malaysian foods do tend to be rather sweet. If I am going somewhere like this I either have a dry, rice-based dish such as nasi goreng (but this does still contain a sweet sauce) or a cha han or some veggies that come more sautéed than drowned in sauce.

◆ Most Indian food, including takeaways, is not usually massively healthy for many reasons (the food often contains lots of fat, colourings and additives, which most of us already know), so if you have to have one, try to choose something dry. I tend to go for the dry chicken tikka as a main (it's just marinated chicken cooked on a skewer with no sauce), and either make or ask for a raita (mint yoghurt dip). If they don't deliver brown rice, I just stick a pan on when I order and it's ready when the meal arrives.

◆ In a Japanese restaurant there are quite a few options, one of the worst being sushi. Instead go for sashimi (which is the fish without the rice) and ask for some brown rice on the side if they can do it.

◆ Italian is also hard because a lot of the dishes – pizza, pasta, white rice – are on the high side of the GI scale, which means they quickly turn to sugar inside the body, but often you'll find a grill on the menu at a good trattoria. Either have that or a salad if your willpower holds out. Otherwise you may have to just go for pasta with the lightest sauce you can find (I like a vongole) and get back on it in the morning.

Takeaways

Most of us know that if we're watching what we eat, a takeaway isn't the best choice. Sometimes, however, there is little choice in the matter. Of all the takeaways you can get, I normally try to go for an Indian and have the dry chicken tikka with brown rice and a raita, as I mentioned above. It's low in fat and sauce, which is important, but it still tastes good. Chinese or Italian takeaways are some of the hardest menus on which to find healthy things. From a Chinese takeaway, try to choose a veggie dish that comes with little sauce. Delivery pizzas from big chains are often high in fat, wheat (high GI) and salt and probably should be avoided if possible.

Going out for drinks

We're all human and there are going to be times when you are going to want to go out for a drink. When this is me, I normally opt for either a glass of nice red wine or a vodka and soda with a big squeeze of fresh lime juice. A dry red wine is not particularly high in sugar and contains lots of antioxidants, namely polyphenols and resveratrol, which are contained in the skins of the grapes. Polyphenols help to keep the body's arteries free from blockages and guard against heart disease and resveratrol has been shown to lower cholesterol). Now I'm no wine buff, but it's thought that pinot noir from cold climates (Chile, Oregon in the USA) contains the most resveratrol because the grape is a difficult variety to grow in cold conditions, meaning it produces lots of antioxidants to protect itself against the frost. Indeed, most red wine grown in cold climates contains more antioxidants than wines grown in warm conditions, so there's a top tip for when you're next perusing a wine list. But, sadly, that can't be too often. Make sure this is just a once in a while treat – there are about 180 calories in each glass of wine, so go easy. If I'm going out with friends who are drinking cocktails, a single vodka, fresh lime and soda is my other fall-back drink. It's known in some circles as a 'skinny b***h' because each serving contains between 80 and 100 calories for a single measure (vodka is between 55 and 90 calories for a shot, the soda water is calorie free and then the rest depends on how much lime you add). Steer clear of beer as, it generally has a high carbohydrate content because of the way the yeast in it is metabolised.

You'll notice that the key element linking most of these choices and options is planning. And planning really is the key to success if you are going to go low sugar.

Be prepared

◆ Always make sure you have a store cupboard full of herbs, spices and whatever else you need to make a quick, healthy meal. I like to ensure I always have eggs, feta and spinach in my fridge as I know that with those three things I can make a breakfast, lunch or dinner if needs be.

◆ Practise your recipes and get to know your quick favourites that you can whip up when you're time poor midweek. Making a tasty frittata is not only healthier than ordering a takeaway or heating up a ready meal, it's quicker too.

◆ Never go to the supermarket when you're hungry. If you find looking at all those old foods you used to buy too tempting, shop online instead.

◆ Always carry healthy snacks with you so you're not caught short on the go.

◆ If you are going out for dinner, try to book a restaurant in advance that has things on the menu that you want to eat. Then you can book a steak house instead of a curry house.

◆ If your mornings are fraught, make more dinner the night before, stick it in the fridge and just put it in your bag in the morning before you leave. Then that's lunch sorted.

◆ Again, if you are pressed for time, try making food in batches and either refrigerating or freezing it – depending what it is, obviously. I do this with breakfasts, such as the protein pancakes (see page 188), or Holly's buckwheat and chia seed brekkie (see page

187). From time to time – when I am feeling especially rock and roll – I make up my own muesli using alternative cereals like spelt, buckwheat and the like and combine it with nuts, seeds, fresh blueberries and whatever else I have in the fridge. Then it's ready to go whenever I need a quick breakfast or a little snack.

The other big change I have made in my life – which I know is easier said than done – is to reduce my stress levels. Stress and sugar have quite an interconnected relationship. Earlier on in the book I explained that eating sugar makes us stressed, but it's also what our bodies biochemically crave when we have been through a period of pressure. If you're one of the many who tend to gain excess weight around the middle (welcome to the club) you need to read on because this concerns you.

As Holly explained earlier, the main reason fat collects around our bellies is because of the stress hormone cortisol. Millions of years ago, our bodies were designed to be able to react very quickly to signs of danger – today we call this the 'fight or flight' response. When your brain thinks your body is in danger, when it gets those stress signals, it releases the hormones adrenaline and cortisol to help you react immediately. This gives you a short burst of energy (glucose from your fat stores) to enable you to get away from whatever threat you are facing. In the olden days, this would have helped you try to outrun a lion or a bear. Today, however, this energy is released almost constantly as a reaction to looming deadlines, the massive electricity bill, traffic jams, the inability to find a parking space and so on... The majority of modern life's stresses and challenges involve hardly using any energy (when was the last time you had to outrun a bear?). So, what does the body do with all that excess energy? It lays it down as fat.

A side effect of the release of the stress hormone cortisol is hunger. We've evolved to have to take in more energy after exerting ourselves so we crave energy-dense foods – sugar and other carbohydrates. You can see how this is going to end up.

Every single person reading this book knows stress isn't good for them. I knew it, yet until a year ago I still lived in a completely stressful environment. Then I left my job and, instead of taking another somewhere else, I struck out on my own. Sometimes it is still panic inducing, but less frequently.

While I loathe it when fortunate people bleat on about leaving their stressful jobs I mention it because, in my defence, I am still the only person paying my whopping mortgage. I'm not from a rich family, and the only income I have is the money I earn. I know that I am fortunate in that my profession allows me to work flexibly and yours may not, but making your life less stressful doesn't have to be as major as leaving your job.

Indeed, for a year before I did leave, I gradually introduced other strategies to try and make my life calmer, such as making time for the things that I enjoy. I completely fell in love with going to the gym again and went back to swimming – something I haven't done much of since I was in my teens. I spend the money I save by not boozing but on seeing a personal trainer at least once a week. While I don't run for hours on the treadmill, I try to do a bit of cardio, then do my own resistance work or take a class in pilates, for example. I made more time to see my friends and family by stopping seeing people that made my life less enjoyable. Each morning I'd get up an hour earlier than I needed to so I could stop rushing to places. I sought help to overhaul my finances and learnt how to politely say 'no' rather than putting myself under never-ending amounts of pressure by over-committing myself.

All of these things helped me stick to my low-sugar plan. If you're ever having a tough time, think about the words at the beginning of this book, 'when you think about giving up, remember why you began'. The best motivation for me has always been thinking back to how I felt – and looked – in 2012. There's no way I want to return to that.

I suppose what I am trying to say is being low sugar doesn't have to be boring or in some way punitive. It's actually a bit of a luxury and a treat. It is time to move away from this idea that people who drink loads of booze and eat lots of rubbish are in some way cool, or that it's somehow exciting. Several experts have already – controversially – likened the sugar industry to the tobacco industry, and look how that has turned out: a ban on smoking in workplaces, public buildings and transportation – not to mention the suggestion that soon, people won't be able to smoke in their own cars if they are driving children somewhere. No one thinks smoking is cool anymore. Some people think it's completely unacceptable. I'm sure in a few years we'll feel the same way about things that are loaded with sugar. You and me, we're just ahead of the curve.

Chapter Eight

A LOW-SUGAR LIFE AND RELATIONSHIPS

This book has told you rather a lot about me: about my body, about what sugar did to my body, my mind and my personality. I've asked you to think about what sugar does to your body, mind and your personality, too. But have you ever thought about what it does to your relationships? How what you eat links you to other people, how it impacts upon your friendships, your family relations and your love life? I hadn't, until I gave it up.

Giving yourself a lifestyle overhaul is as empowering as it is isolating. Because I got a lot of my emotional validation from sweet food – I turned to it when I had a bad day, for example, or leant on it when someone had let me down – jettisoning it initially left me feeling as if I had a bit of a void in my life. I was expecting it, and I also knew from reading other people's experiences that it would be short lived. Indeed, the feeling disappeared in a few short weeks when I trained myself to stop seeing food as a reward.

What I wasn't expecting, however, were some of the reactions from people I knew and cared about. While not being outright unsupportive, many muttered the words 'life's too short!' whenever we went out for dinner or drinks and I chose something that didn't meet with their approval: a glass of fizzy water instead of a cocktail, for instance; grilled fish and salad instead of a pizza; a peppermint tea instead of a dessert.

Over recent months I have talked about being low sugar to quite a lot of people. It's a hot topic in the media right now, so people are generally curious as to how I started, how I maintain it and the like. But back then, in the beginning, I hardly told anyone that I was trying to cut out most forms of sugar. I didn't want to, in case I failed. I certainly didn't sit down at a dinner and look at other people's plates longingly, or bemoan all of the things on the menu that I couldn't eat, which would invite comment. Indeed, I rarely said anything at all unless people noticed.

Yet a few people – and I must stress it was very few but they were rather vociferous – would berate me at the table for 'being so restrictive'. Some told me that I wasn't choosing what I '*wanted* to eat' but instead, choosing what I 'thought I *should* eat' because it was more healthy – as if I couldn't *want* to choose something healthy for my own dinner. These are people who are not ignorant about health and looking after yourself, yet they made me feel as if I were failing them by choosing something relatively unindulgent. It was a form of competitive eating – something I've not experienced before. And it was most odd.

My not often drinking is another obvious bone of contention for many people. This won't come as a surprise to many of you. We've all attended parties where we've not drunk for some reason but been badgered all evening to do so. Nights at the pub appeared to be rather tainted – for friends – if I didn't drink. Which was ironic because it often makes no difference to me. To keep the peace, I admit I will sometimes order a soda water and ask the bartender to stick a slice of lime in it so I can tell people it's a vodka, lime and soda.

I can't fathom why it is socially acceptable for someone to go on about a friend abstaining from something, when it wouldn't be socially acceptable for me to comment on the reverse. For example, it would be frowned upon for me to pipe up to the person sitting next to me at dinner and say 'Why are you ordering something so unhealthy? Is it that you don't like yourself very much?' Or, similarly 'It's interesting to me that you see high-sugar, high-fat, high-carbohydrate food as a "treat". Why do you think this is?'

Everyone would, quite rightly, think me rude as hell and a total pain in the arse.

I asked London-based psychologist and writer Amanda Hills, who specialises in addictions and behaviour change, why she thinks our efforts at self-improvement are sometimes met negatively by people who care about us.

'You are right when you say that commenting on someone's "unhealthy" choice is less socially acceptable than saying something about someone's "healthy" choice,' she says. 'People often find themselves the subject of criticism or judgment if they abstain from something, you know the "just have a pudding, life's too short" brigade. Yet, it would be unfathomable for people to make a similar snide comment to someone who was eating a deep fried Brie for example. Few people would say "have a beef burger, live a little" to a vegetarian because they respect it as a life choice. It's often not the case with giving up something like sugar,'

Jane (the friend I mentioned in some earlier chapters) has been ultra supportive towards my sugar-free lifestyle, and she has an interesting theory on why some people take exception when another makes a life change, whether that's the type of clothes they wear, the type of music they listen to or the sort of food that they eat.

'Maybe it's because we're all drawn to people who are similar to us in some way, that we have something in common with,' she says. 'Commonality is one of the unofficial laws of attraction. When you appear to stop liking something you used to like, or that you liked when you met someone, perhaps it subconsciously makes them suspicious in some way? It's as if you have "changed".'

So, why did this happen? Was it out of concern or, like Jane says, fear of change? Because others thought I was holding a mirror up to what they perceive to be their failngs? Or was it competition? I'm many things, but I'm not a competitive person. I don't really care what anyone else does, says, eats or wears. I've kind of always moved to the beat of my own drum. For instance, if I wanted cake and no one else did, I would order the cake. In fact, that's how I ended up having to cut back on sugar in the first place, but I digress.

'Food is the major form of social bonding,' says Amanda. 'It doesn't just start when we go out to dinners with friends, it starts very early, from our experiences with our parents. Obviously we're fed by our mother when we're born and even before that in the womb.'

But is there something bonding about indulging in 'special foods' – you know, the things we often deem 'treats'? Perhaps there's a sense that, if you don't get involved, you're somehow distancing yourself from the sense of celebration? Amanda thinks so.

'Sweet things are considered to be "a treat" because human beings have evolved to like them. Eating them has a positive effect on our brain and causes it to release dopamine and serotonin. Therefore, as we grow, when people want to express love, they often do it in the form of sweets and sweet things or candy because they know it gives the other person pleasure. This is a pretty universal culture the world over. If you choose not to get involved in that, it can cause a reaction in people.'

In other words, people can become suspicious of your actions or even negative towards you.

'I have spent many years researching, working with patients and anecdotally talking to friends about why this is and I believe that people's negative reactions to someone else's abstinence from something or other – whether that's sugar or something else like smoking – is because it threatens them,' says Amanda.

'It's very common because it means they then have to look at their own behaviour. Quite often you'll find that the person who makes a negative comment has tried to give up something themselves, but hasn't managed to. I normally find that they would like to quit too, but they're either not in the right place mentally or they have tried to quit before and failed and they're not ready to try again. Their way of trying to impose some control over it themselves is by criticising, or appearing to judge, someone who is managing to do it. It makes them feel better about their own failure. Criticism can sometimes come from a good and genuine place. Perhaps it could be that someone likes you and genuinely wants you to enjoy yourself, but that's not the case with sugar. We all know that too much of it is not a good thing...

'You rarely get someone who has achieved what they want to – be that stopping smoking, cutting back on drinking, eating more healthily or whatever it is – passing judgment on someone else who is trying to make a change.'

I think we probably all have a friend who fits Amanda's description. My lowest point with a pal was when we went to a wedding together – sharing a room – last year. It was a long-weekend affair, starting on the Thursday evening and ending on a Sunday afternoon. There's no other way to describe her reaction to my eating and drinking habits over the three days than massive disappointment. I'd obviously been tagged as her partner in food and drink crimes and she reacted to my not toeing the line as if I'd somehow duped her or buddied up with her under false pretenses. Said friend spent the best part of the weekend trying to pressure me into eating things I didn't want to – afternoon teas, big bits of cake, glasses of champagne in quick succession, puddings etc. – not because there was nothing else to eat, but because she wanted to eat them and, presumably didn't want to do so alone. It was very tiring. When I didn't buckle and give in, she appeared a little bit annoyed, as if my choices were affecting her enjoyment of the festivities. Yet I was still enjoying the nuptials – being outgoing, cutting some shapes on the dance floor, and staying up until a respectable hour – all the things I would normally do at a wedding. I was perplexed by her reaction to my lifestyle, and surprised, mainly because I've been friends with this person for many years and I know she cares deeply about me and my wellbeing, and the feeling is mutual. So, how to explain her behavior?

'What you're talking about is effectively an attempt at sabotage,' says Amanda, 'and sabotage is very interesting. People do attempt to sabotage other people's lifestyle changes and this is normally because there's something about themselves that they don't feel good about. For example, some people have friends who encourage them to drink more than they want to. Getting a second bottle of wine together makes the friend feel that their choice has been validated.

'What happens when you go against that – say you don't have the extra glass of wine, or you choose not to eat a pudding – is that you are threatening your friend's whole idea of what is "okay". It forces them to look at their behaviour and their choices, which is uncomfortable.'

I also wonder if I perhaps fulfilled a specific role in people's lives. Before cutting back on sugar, I was the bon viveur, slightly chubby, funny friend who didn't really give a damn whether what I was eating or drinking was in some way indulgent. When I left women's magazines to start working at a newspaper back in 2003, I was quickly indoctrinated into the practice of getting a bottle of wine, some crisps or maybe some chips and mayonnaise most nights at the pub after work. Obviously this did my waistline no favours, but it did make me rather lively company to be around of an evening.

'We often have a "role" in the lives of others,' says Amanda. 'Whether we have created that role through some of our past behaviours or whether it's a role that other people have put on us because it's where they feel most comfortable having us, for some reason. A lot of this has to do with positions in a social group – frequently someone becomes known as the picky one, there's the person who plays the role of the party animal, perhaps a slightly shy person, then a flaky friend who always says she'll come out and cancels at the last minute... These are just examples, but if you think about your friendship group, you'll often notice each person has a part that they play. If you are changing and evolving – and most of us want to evolve in some way, and not be the same person we were five years ago – it's a threat to someone else. It means they have to hold a mirror up to themselves, to take a look at themselves and think "actually I'm not sure I'm that happy with what I've got". There's also an element of competition between women about food that men don't seem to have so much.'

I asked Ian Marber where he feels sweet food gets its symbolism from, when in reality it is just a simple fuel.

'Sugar and food is dumbed down. We live in a society where everything is dumbed down. Food is described as "yummy" or "naughty" or a "treat", which is quite a puerile way to think about it.

There is a childish fetishised notion around sweet things too. Cupcakes are a perfect example. I always wonder if the fascination with these things is a hangover from childhood because they look like something you'd find at a dolly's tea party. They're pretty, they're colourful and cute, they're like a young girl's version of a food.

I've always thought they were disgusting, but there's something about them that's 'pretty' and *'Sex and the City'*-ish, it's as if they're a fashionable accessory, and I say fashionable because they are everywhere. Cupcake shops exist in glamorous areas of London where people don't eat any carbohydrates, let alone sugar. I'm not sure where this demand comes from. There is something about sharing 'treat' food that is bonding. You can't imagine the guys at *Men's Health* magazine sitting around asking each other if they would like a cupcake. It's comical. Yet that is exactly what happens in women's magazine offices.'

Talking of men, let's discuss the terrifying subject of sober dating. It's long been my opinion that meeting someone new is nerve-wracking enough without the need for it to be done sober. Yet when I started my low-sugar life I was single. Dating while drinking was hard enough, I couldn't bear to think about what dating without drinking was going to be like. It was one of my main reservations about starting this whole thing. I have a single female friend who rarely drinks and entertains us all with amazingly unattractive stories of heinous dates with men who get rather too drunk, rather too fast. We've all spent evenings being bored by inebriated people while we're sober. There's nothing like it to make you want to go home to bed – on your own, which isn't something many of us crave, long term.

In the summer of 2012, I was a fairly happy lone-ranger, with no one waiting in the wings to alter that status. Although Mum, through Natalie, my sister, was determined I should go internet dating (argh) I'd decided that I wanted to get myself sorted out – by which I mean getting comfortable with this new regime of mine, getting a bit fitter and trying to balance my skin – before I would ride the merry-go-round of love again. I couldn't sleep with a face covered in Sudocrem at the start of a new relationship, unless I wanted it to be the end of a new relationship. No, when all of those things had been taken care of, then I would turn my attention to matters of the heart.

But then matters of the heart were taken out of my hands.

One warm afternoon in September 2012, I felt the familiar sensation of my phone humming in my dress pocket. I'd slipped out of work for an hour to go to the hairdresser in an oh-so-posh part of west London and imagined it was work summoning me back before I'd even got to my appointment. Thank God it wasn't. It was a text reading: 'Who the hell is James Smith?'.

My stomach lurched. Those six words spelled trouble. Barry was back.

Barry isn't his real name. Thankfully.

At 35, Barry was a couple of years older than me, and worked in the City. We'd initially met a year before in the summer of 2011 at a work event. We talked, I liked him but he had to leave to go on to something else. Even though we only spoke for about 20 minutes, Bazza had made quite an impression on me. He behaved like he owned the party, not in a loud way, but he was incredibly alpha and quietly confident. The next day at work, I kept talking about him to friends. They, quite rightly, told me to stop talking and start acting (being quite shy and terrified of rejection, it's not something I'm good at). But as he'd told me his name, I tracked him down on Facebook and asked him out for a drink.

While waiting for his reply, I checked in on Facebook approximately every 15 minutes. I even woke up in the night and checked it. Nothing. The next night, while riding the bus home, I got a Facebook alert. Just when I'd almost given up on him, Barry had replied. We arranged to go for a 'cup of tea' a few weeks later when I got back from holiday in Bali.

It was, literally, a cup of tea. Shock horror, Barry didn't drink. He's not a recovering alcoholic, but he doesn't like alcohol and, as such, has been tee-total for quite a few years.

I was taken aback. Finding a man in London who doesn't drink is like successfully panning for gold in the Thames. At the time, I was quite into my cocktails and wasn't sure I could relax in the company of a man who pointedly abstained. We met up quite a few times in a 'getting to know you' way but I never felt Barry was that keen, which was a shame as I thought he was the bees knees. Tall, handsome, funny, geeky, successful, clever, solvent, argumentative. We liked the same films and music. We both loved Chevy Chase. I like to be independent and do my own thing, so does Barry. Like me, he was close to his family and into having adventures. He lived fairly nearby in his own flat and was well travelled – he'd frequently regale me with stories about scrapes he'd gotten himself into. He was excellent with money and, without being patronising, he tried to sort out my chaotic spending habits – which was something I was in desperate need of. Basically, Barry had everything I liked, and I wasn't at all swung by the fact that he, excitingly, had a car (a rarity in central London) and drove everywhere.

Then, as abruptly as it began, Barry disappeared. We saw each other early in the afternoon on New Year's Eve 2011 – we were both going to pre-arranged separate parties. In January, I texted him a few times, trying to play it cool, but he'd rarely reply and if I ever asked a question or suggested hanging out, he'd go silent.

I bemoaned his loss to colleagues on an almost daily basis. I'd really liked Barry, so much that I'd even turned a blind eye to my normal deal-breakers, namely that he wore bad shoes and often terrible jeans, followed Frankie Boyle on Twitter (yuk, why?) and had a fondness for taking his phone out and going onto Facebook in the middle of a conversation. Yes, he was a bit lazy, driving around and then sitting on my sofa while I ran around waiting on him, but I felt like he could be my partner in crime – the Terry to my June, the Shaggy to my Scooby-Doo, the Siegfried to my Roy… you get the idea. Plus, I was desperate to get my hands on his wardrobe and have a good old clear-out.

But Barry was gone and I had to move on. The new year came around and while I often thought of him and wondered if I'd done something to cause him to disappear from my life so abruptly – especially because I thought we got on so well, even just on a friend level – I was determined not to go into 2012 mourning someone who patently didn't want to be with me and, worse still, didn't have the balls to explain why. At the end of spring I began spending a lot of time with a friend of a friend called Chris, the bon viveur I talked about in Chapter One.

I wasn't sure where, if anywhere, this one was going, but we were eating and drinking a lot while finding out, which was obviously fun. Sunday roasts with a bottle of good wine – then maybe a couple of extra glasses on top – were a regular thing. Then, there were desserts. There were always desserts. Crème brûlées with that delectable layer of crisp toasted sugar, or a hot chocolate pudding, light as air with a centre of thick, oozing molten cocoa. As I was a big (and getter bigger) ice cream fan, I would be sure to layer a couple of scoops onto whichever pudding would allow it. At home, a few hours later, there would be toasted teacakes and crumpets with jam for tea and maybe another glass or two of wine. While it was fun, Mondays, understandably, were often met with bleary eyes and a fuzzy head – not an ideal way to start a gruelling week at work. Although I tried to be healthy whenever I wasn't with him – which was the majority of the week because he had a tough job in banking – my clothes were getting tighter. I began living in my smock dresses rather than my bodycon ones. This was when I bought the stunning little number for my birthday party in May from Dolce & Gabbana… in a size 16. Not a good sign.

After a couple of months, Chris and I realised it would be best if we remained friends rather than anything more. It was the right move, but I was still nursing wounded pride. Everyone wants someone to fight for them, or to make a grand gesture, like writing them a power ballad or commandeering a billboard to proclaim how they couldn't cope if you left them. Instead, I'd been let go of with something of a whimper, using the dreaded 'shall we just be friends' line, which everyone knows really means 'I just don't fancy you very much'. Sigh.

I was despondent to again be back at 'Go' on the Monopoly Board of Love and sought solace at the gym – something I have always relied upon to regulate my emotions. I find nothing ever feels as bad after you've spent 45 minutes making yourself pointlessly hot and bothered. Often I'm just overwhelmed with relief that I've survived.

The next week, in a pique of self-improvement, I started my low-sugar life. For the first time in months, I stopped caring about not having a love interest and instead concentrated on looking after myself. I felt even-keeled for the first time in a while. Things were going well.

But then Barry returned, out of the blue. It was his trademark style: curt, rather alpha-male, not asking how I was, not apologising for behaving like an idiot and hurting my feelings, not explaining why he'd been absent for months. Nope, the message merely asked me if I knew who someone was.

I waited for about, ooohh, ten seconds before replying, 'Hello, Barry. Nice to hear from you. I'm very well. Thanks for asking', and pressed send. Sod him, asking me a question out of the blue without even any pre-amble. While I knew who James Smith was (the boyfriend of a mutual friend), why should I tell him? A big part of me hoped he wouldn't reply, as I didn't know if I could handle riding another love roller-coaster, even though I did look hot – slimmer and tanned from my Spanish break. A couple of minutes later, he replied. 'Ha ha' he said and explained he was in Poland for a client.

So that was it then, he must have been bored.

We exchanged flirty badinage and decided to see each other when he returned a few weeks later.

While I didn't want to be, I was excited. I loved his company and the prospect of seeing him, even as friends, was another reason to be strict with myself. One night a few weeks later, he came over for food. I'd been spending my copious evenings in over the past few months trying out new healthy recipes and re-learning how to cook, so I took real pride in some of my new healthy creations.

Barry's an athletic-looking guy but he must have hollow legs because he can sure put food away. From my healthy curries with brown rice to marinated fillet steak with spinach salad and chicken and cashew nut stir-fries, he ate anything I put in front of him. I've always loved to look after someone and Barry let me.

And of course, Barry didn't drink. There were no evenings spent in the pub, no after-work rendezvous at a bar in town, no pressure to 'go on, just have one'. We normally met up at my house, where we'd sit, listen to music and just hang out. Sometimes we'd go for dinner, but often, it was just him and me (and the iPad, always the bloody iPad) and it was great. I felt like I had a new best friend. In the beginning, he was a sugar monster, chomping his way through large bars of Green & Black's or pieces of cake, but after about a year Barry stopped eating so much sugar too. He ditched the chocolate he was so fond of in favour of plain yoghurt with toasted almonds and cinnamon for pudding. I hasten to say that it was a gradual thing and under no encouragement from me. And you know what boys are like with food, one minute I'd see him eating two almond croissants for breakfast, then the next I'd be listening to him drone on about him being low-sugar. Yet Barry's acceptance of my own food choices was one of the many reasons I was so besotted with him, and one of the main factors that kept me to my new way of eating.

Which is really the whole reason I am mentioning Barry. Firstly, it's to show that, even though after 18 months it didn't work out between us, it is possible to meet someone great, even when you're not doing the whole 'going to bars, getting drunk and accosting a stranger' thing that most of us are used to doing on the dating scene. Of course, I was helped because Barry didn't drink, but my time with him taught me that the whole dating-nerves thing doesn't have to be overcome by getting blotto. Secondly, it's because without Barry, I'm not sure my sugar-free pact would have lasted. He came along just at the right time to help me through what could have been a tough patch. Regardless of the ups and downs between us – and there were many – he never put temptation in my way. When I made Barry my trademark melty chocolate brownies he never asked me to eat one, perhaps because he's undoubtedly endured years of people whining on at him to have a drink when he didn't want to. When we were away on holiday in the States for a couple of weeks, he ordered pancake stacks pretty much every day, covering them in a dusting of icing sugar, strawberries, then maple syrup. Unlike many, Barry never tried to force-feed me a delicious mouthful to show me what I was missing or convince me to indulge.

Despite his failings – and he'd be the first to admit that he has a quite a few – Barry made my unusual eating habits feel normal and for that I will always be grateful.

Because, if you want to make lasting life changes like cutting back on sweet stuff, I can't stress enough the importance of having a 'Barry'. Your Barry has to look out for you, to be your best friend and support you in whatever decisions you make about cutting back on sugar, whether that's to stay in and turn into a hermit, to not tell anyone what you're doing or to broadcast it to the world and become an evangelist. Ideally they'll go along for the ride too, but if not, they just have to not hinder your journey. It's as simple as that.

I've also found other mentors along the way. Although I started seeing Holly Pannett just a few months into my low-sugar lifestyle, she's become a friend. During our once-weekly personal training sessions, we talk about life, work, love and nutrition. I've learnt so much from her, including that it's important not to be too uptight about what you do and don't eat. She understands what I am trying to achieve and has supported me all the way.

Last year I also met James Duigan, the author of the *Clean and Lean* books, who invited me to his Bodyism gym to meet some of his personal trainers and work out. It was all rather life-changing. Here was a gym full of kind, beautiful healthy people, all of whom follow the principles of James' Clean and Lean programme. Spending time with them gave me a sense of community, it enabled me to see that there were lots of people out there who believed the same things I did, and that it wasn't somehow strange to be doing what I'm doing.

But, as I mentioned earlier, it's going to be pretty tough to completely overhaul your life if you are faced with resistance from your nearest and dearest.

'Critcising people for being healthy is a very cultural thing,' says Amanda. 'It's something that seems to happen explicitly, but probably not exclusively, in this country. I've just come back from America and – while of course it's not the same in all parts of the country – if you explained to people in Los Angeles or New York that you'd cut back on sugar, it would be applauded. Not so in London. The English mindset lags very far behind on things like this; it's not in our national psyche to encourage people to get healthy. The only time it seems to be accepted is if you have a reason to be – for example if you're an athlete. Otherwise, being seen to be putting effort into being healthy taps into this national dislike we have of people who "try too hard". It goes against the English way. It's almost as if we enjoy it when people have a problem with something. If someone does well on a diet, quite often you'll hear comments along the lines of "yes, but have you seen how skinny she's got?"'

I've already talked about how overhauling your diet also goes hand in hand with a complete lifestyle change, and part of that was changing how I see my friends socially.

While this possibly sounds like the most virtuous thing in the world, I quite often arrange to go to exercise classes with some of my nearest and dearest. Katy and I have been to yoga and pilates classes together. Whereas we used to spend evenings sitting in an old man's pub opposite her house. Jane and I sometimes now play tennis. Seafront walks have replaced grotty pub crawls around Brighton with my school-friend Julie. Maya and I have dinema evenings, where we'll go out for dinner and the cinema instead of tearing it up around east London. Food and drink is still a major and important component of my life, but now there are other things too.

Of course, part of this comes with getting older. In your mid-thirties you stop wanting to be the oldest person in a club. Waking up with a hangover isn't something that just fades away before lunchtime, it's a whole-day event (maybe even two). Most of my friends now have young children, which means nights out are less frequent. If they want a big one, they're probably not going to call me – at least not me alone – to be their partner in crime anymore, but that doesn't mean I don't see them.

While people do often say to me 'oh, are you *still* doing that low-sugar thing?' when we are out at dinner, as if – after two years and all the articles I have written about my decision – it would just be a passing phase, they rarely pressure me or ask me to explain why I am doing it. I guess once you start looking and feeling healthier, the reasons are pretty obvious to see.

So, what are the best ways to cope when someone is being unsupportive? Amanda had this to say:

> 'When someone is trying to persuade you to do something that is not going to be beneficial for you, I almost want to ask them if they're scared of giving something up themselves.'

For example, if someone was trying to convince me to eat a cake, I could turn around and say 'I think you'd like to give up sugar, but you are too scared'. If you don't think you can handle taking such a confrontational approach, Amanda does have three tips that may help you to deal with friends or loved ones who have difficulty accepting or adapting to your change.

> 'There are three levels of dealing with people who are unsupportive,' Amanda says. 'Level one is for acquaintances, people who aren't your close friends but that you do socialise with. If you are out with them or see them and feel they've judged you or your choices harshly, I recommend simply saying something along the lines of "I have chosen to do this at the moment, I don't really want to go into the ins

and outs of why tonight as we're in a social situation, but I'd be very happy to talk to you about it another time if you're really interested". You don't need to be especially stern about it, do it with a smile, but say it with conviction.

'Level two is for close friends. If you find they aren't being as nice as they could be about whatever it is you are trying to achieve, whether that's giving up sugar or giving up smoking, approach them one-on-one. Say to them "can I tell you what is going on with me and why I am doing this?" Once you have sat down with them and had an honest and open conversation, explaining what you want to achieve, whether that's feeling healthier, losing weight, changing your skin, whatever it is, you'll find most people are incredibly supportive. If they're still not, once you have told them the reasons, you may need to think about whether you want to maintain the friendship and if they have your best interests at heart. Friends really should respect your decisions – especially when they're well thought out, intelligent ones, like making a change to benefit your health.

'Level three is reserved for the people you live with. If you're not finding them supportive, you may have to explain why you're doing what you're doing more than once, and explain why it's important to you. It's key to remember that when you are trying to change you can only change yourself. You can't change other people. Also, if the other person is resistant, you won't change their mindset overnight. The only way to proceed is by being consistent and firm. Try not to get emotional or tearful when talking about it or explaining your reasoning. If you are trying to make a change and it's hard for your family or partner to cope with, you need to say "this is what I have decided to do for me" and remind them that you are an adult capable of making your own decisions. Remind people that you are fully equipped to make your own life choices and as part of that you are taking responsibility for what you do to yourself. All you are asking in return is for them to respect it. Remember though, you may have to have these conversations a few times until it sinks in.'

If you have children, the issue is slightly more complicated, and, Amanda says, needs to be dealt with sensitively.

'I'd advise someone who was trying to cut back on sugar not to go into the ins and outs, the whys and wherefores of their decision if they have kids,' she says. 'Definitely do not demonise sugar or make it into a big deal. Food is just food and that should be the message. It's just fuel. Treats shouldn't have emotions attached to them, but quite a lot of the time they do.

The only way to deal with this is to try and strike a balance. Healthy behaviour around food means not demonising anything at all and being moderate. If you are discussing it, always come from the health point of view, never from the looks side of things. Educating your children about which food is healthy and why is of course a good thing, but try not to use the word "bad". Instead use the words "healthy choices" and "less healthy choices"'.

Even with the best willpower in the world and all the support you could possibly want, there are going to be times that when you find it hard to stick to your new regime. In the next chapter I'm going to tell you how to get your head in the right place to stick with your new low-sugar lifestyle.

Chapter Nine

MAINTAINING A LOW-SUGAR LIFE

Yesterday, I sat in a café in a well-to-do part of London and ate scrambled eggs, smoked salmon and mushrooms while I watched the world go by. I was meant to be writing this book, but had decided to take a break, go to the gym and then have some lunch. The weather was glorious. Britons were emerging from their houses, blinking into the sunlight like moles coming out from their burrows after a long winter.

As I hopelessly procrastinated – as I am wont to do – a woman came in and sat down at the table next to me. In front of us at a table in the window were laid a plethora of brownies, treacle tarts, meringues and several large cakes. I didn't look at them too intently, for obvious reasons. When the server came over, the lady next to me said she was waiting for a friend and would catch her eye when she arrived, which she duly did. The server came back and tried to take their order. After requesting their drinks, the friend who arrived first asked the latecomer if she'd like to get a cake. The latecomer said no, she was watching what she ate because she was going on holiday at Easter. The first friend pressed on, undaunted: 'do you want to share something then?' she asked. The latecomer again said she didn't think so, no. The first friend tutted, muttered the immortal words 'oh, I'll feel bad ordering a whole thing. Let's share a small brownie.' At which point, the dieting friend acquiesced, beaten down by the domineering feeder she was meeting who wouldn't take two firm 'no's for an answer.

I note this because learning how to say 'no' and staying on the wagon are what this chapter is all about. There are a lot of 'treats' out there. Cakes, biscuits, crisps, flavoured yoghurts, chocolate bars, fizzy drinks, alcohol, fruit, smoothies, milkshakes, pasta, ice cream, white rice, sweeteners, bread, ketchup, baked beans, pastries, one lump or two, ready meals, dried fruit, honey, cereals, puddings, sweets, sauces, cordials, takeaway coffees, muesli bars, ready-made sandwiches, takeaways, agave, pizza, preserves and chutneys...

These are just some of the ones I can think of. All different forms but with one thing in common, they all sound delicious. If you're reading this in Britain, I'm sure you're nodding – we consume almost six million litres of sugary drinks every year. Then there's chocolate – research suggests Britons ate between 9.5 kg and 11 kg of chocolate per capita in 2012. In other words, we guzzled over 211 standard-sized bars each, in a year. This made us the third largest consumers of chocolate in the world, behind Switzerland and Ireland.

While it's horrible to have to cut out something you enjoy, you're going to have to stop eating this kind of stuff as often as you do. As I've already mentioned, it's not just me saying it, the World Health Organization is almost certainly going to recommend we all halve our intakes of sugar later this year. They believe it's making us fatter and sicker, and rotting our teeth. Significantly scaling back our intake is the only way to change ourselves.

I know you're not looking forward to it. Few sane people embrace the idea of depriving themselves. Even faced with all the advantages that cutting back on sugar will bring to your life, it's a hard path to tread. It means deferring your pleasures from the short term to the long term. Abstaining from the fruit juice and cereals you like in the morning to have better skin in three months. These are the very real choices you face.

Many psychologists believe that making a change happens in stages. Each of us goes through these phases – I know I did – before we decide whether to implement healthy improvements into our lives.

'There is a model for change, and it can apply to any change that you make,' says Amanda Hills. 'Over 30 years ago, two alcoholism researchers Carlo Di Clemente and J.O. Prochaska noticed that people who wanted to alter something about their life all went through these stages before they tried to alter their behaviour, which is why it's called the Stages of Change model.

'The first stage is called pre-contemplation' says Amanda. 'Here's an example. I used to be a very light smoker, then I started doing yoga. As part of my practice, I was told to focus on my body and together with deep breathing I started thinking about my lovely lungs and how lucky I was to have such a well-functioning body. Obviously, I knew there was tar in cigarettes, but in my yoga practice I started to picture the tar sitting there in my lungs. My pre-contemplation was "yuk. I don't think I want to smoke any more". For someone who wants to cut back on their sugar intake, they may start thinking about the way sugar is ageing their skin from the inside, our how it's playing havoc with their hormones. Perhaps they'll imagine themselves gaining weight as they age, possibly even getting ill. Pre-contemplation does not mean that you are ready to give up, but it shows an awareness.'

You are obviously already at the pre-contemplation stage, that's why you're reading this book. For me, pre-contemplation happened very quickly. Literally in a matter of hours. I thought about my diet, I realised the amount of sweetness I was consuming and had a lightbulb moment – perhaps the sugar could be contributing to a lot of negative things I was feeling and seeing when I looked in the mirror.

'The second stage is contemplation,' says Amanda 'This is where you sit down and think about the potential change, you wonder what it would it be like if you gave up. This leads to rehearsals in your mind, forming little scenarios and daydreams of how your day would be. You'll wonder how something – in this case, giving up sugar – would work; whether you could do it. With giving up sugar, you subconsciously visualise yourself in a certain situation and wonder "could I be someone who doesn't drink alcohol? Could I be the person who doesn't eat any junk food?". Within this stage comes rehearsal. You'll find yourself almost doing role plays in your mind, thinking about who would be the best people to socialise with, who would tolerate your not drinking the best, who or where you should avoid. For instance, you could find yourself thinking: "well, if I went out with X and Y it would be alright because they don't drink. However if I saw Z it would be more difficult because they're a real party animal".'

Remember my story about being sad I'd never go to the beer festival in Munich, or I'd never sit on the beach with a friend drinking beer? This was a rather melodramatic part of my contemplation stage. It's worth bearing in mind that professionals believe many people wanting to make changes in their life 'rehearse' scenarios in their mind that are much more negative than the reality would ever be. In other words, they underestimate the pros and overestimate the cons. For example, I've already told you I felt sad I wouldn't be able to share a Bikini Blonde on the beach with a friend again. But there's no reason why I couldn't sit on the beach drinking beer with a friend if I really wanted to. Even if I didn't want to drink a beer, I could sit on the beach with a friend and have a memorable, enjoyable time. In 15 drinking years I had between the ages of 18 and 33, when I decided to cut back on sugar, I never attended Munich's Oktoberfest. Probably because I've never really wanted to. Quite why I lamented it in my contemplation phase I don't know.

> 'Stage three is preparation or readiness. This is where you are ready to try. It doesn't mean you're going to succeed first time, in fact, people often don't and they slip up once or even a few times,' says Amanda.

It's thought that being well prepared is one of the secrets to achieving a lasting change in your life. Throwing out all the junk in my cupboards was my preparation phase. I was getting ready to try, removing all the temptations that it was in my power to remove. The next day, however, I rummaged in the bin and drank the dregs of that bottle of cordial. Not exactly a heinous crime and I don't even count it as slipping up, but it was certainly a step on the road to my being ready. Experts say that this phase is where people typically should be encouraged to seek help from friends. This was when I told my friends at work what I was planning to do and they helped me stay on the straight and narrow.

'Then comes action' says Amanda. 'It's a pretty self-explanatory stage. You have taken the steps – so you've quit sugar or given up smoking.'

It's thought that the action phase lasts as long as six months after you've made your change – in this case, cutting back on sugar. Experts believe you should reward yourself often to keep reinforcing that this was a good change to make. The reward for you is, as you cut back on your sugar intake, the newer, healthier version of you starts to emerge. If this is too wholesome for you, do what I've always done; treat yourself to some new bits for your wardrobe. I've always been a big shopper. For my 13th birthday I asked for money and went to Guildford for the day with Natalie, Mum and her friend Chris, who drove us all in her convertible Jeep. I spent almost all of my birthday swag on a pair of Calvin Klein knickers, a matching vest and a Benetton bag. It was a better decision than the one I made on my 12th birthday when I begged my parents to allow me to get my hair permed – something the hairdresser in downtown Worthing duly did – only she included my fringe. It was stunning only in its awfulness.

But yes. If you're really stuck for something to keep you going, go clothes shopping. It doesn't matter if your budget is Primark or Prada, a few new bits and bobs are not only a nice reward but they're also useful because, despite not feeling like you're 'on a diet', your waistline will be shrinking at a weekly rate.

'Lastly comes maintenance,' says Amanda. 'When you get to this stage you have successfully managed to change. You've kept up your new behaviour for a while – banishing all the so-called "treat" foods and modifying your behaviour. Even at this late stage there's still a possibility that you could slip up, since we are all human!'

The maintenance part of the model only really begins after you've passed the six months stage. Even then, experts recommend you steer clear of situations that could put you in the way of temptation – which is rather more easy for some addictions than others. Because high levels of refined sugar are found in the majority of products on the shelves of our supermarkets, even daily chores will put people trying to implement a low-sugar lifestyle in the way of temptation. You know that your body will give up sugar much more easily than your mind. I've already told you that for the first few days of my detox, every time I saw someone drinking a can of Coca-Cola, I had to fight the urge to go up and ask them for a sip. My mind was still repeatedly whirring away, obsessing about sugar long after my body had given up its intense regular cravings for the white stuff, way past when I'd started to notice an increase in my energy levels, far down the line of my gradual weight-loss, and after my skin had begun to improve. It's tough to quash the nagging feeling at the back of your brain that's encouraging you to 'go on, just have the one biscuit' or saying 'a small piece of cake won't make much difference'.

But, you know what? It really doesn't matter if you fall (or jump) off the wagon from time to time. In fact, I think it's better to have and cherish something you really want, give yourself a break and accept it as a rarity.

If you're still eating lots of sugar now and have a fairly substantial dependency, what you'll realise as you travel down your road of lowering your intake is that, sometimes, temptations will spring up from nowhere. When you're least expecting it, you'll round a corner and walk into someone eating a Mint Chocolate Cornetto that will set the corners of your mouth twitching. It happened to me just yesterday when I was in Brighton on a sunny spring day, although I didn't give in. Other times, the urge to eat something sweet will slowly sneak up on you. Perhaps you'll have been dealing with daily pressure from work, family, friends or financial or health worries but, getting on with things, accepting them, not letting them get you down and then bam! You *feel* you need to indulge. It happens to the best of us.

Instead of imposing an unwavering standard upon myself whereby I must *never* have something I desire, I find it helpful to accept that sometimes I may eat something sweet, but that straight afterwards, I'll go back to my healthier way of eating and no real damage will have been done. I always think it's of the utmost importance that you're kind to yourself, pretty much in everything, but especially in this time of change. Be your own best friend. I don't believe in yo-yoing – having one day on something, and one day off (unless it's the 5:2 diet, which seems to work for lots of people but it isn't about cutting one thing out) – and a plan like this definitely wouldn't work with going low sugar simply because it takes a while to eliminate your cravings. That's why I've never set aside a dedicated 'treat' day, as some people do, because I've not really found it helpful to spend a significant amount of time eating the things I used to so enjoy. Indulging over a meal once a fortnight or however often isn't a problem... Once every two days, however? That's rather more of one.

Because even though I have written this book extolling the joys of cutting back my sugar intake, I'm not immune to temptation either. From time to time I'll have a glass of good red wine (organic, if possible, as it usually contains fewer sulphites, which are used to preserve it, but a nice quality one if not). I try to make sure I indulge when I'm in a 'good place', that is, not when I've had a crap day at work or an argument with someone. It took me long enough to scale back my emotional associations with food, and I'm loathe to help them gain a hold over me again.

If I'm out with friends or at a dinner party I will sometimes have a glass of red, for no other reason than I enjoy it. That in itself is a rather liberating way to feel. Likewise it's not the end of the world if you eat a baked Alaska one evening, although after a few weeks being low sugar, the thought of this will be enough to set your teeth on edge, I guarantee it.

When you succumb, which you will do because we aren't robots, what really matters is not dwelling on it, not obsessing over it, and accepting that you haven't 'undone' all the progress that you've made just by having, say, a scoop of ice cream. Don't feel guilty about it – the one thing I hope you have learnt by reading this book is that food should not be emotional. After you've eaten, and importantly, enjoyed whatever sweet thing you chose, go straight back to your low-sugar mindset.

It's not ideal to fall off the wagon and stay off for a few days or more – say, eating sweet things three times a day every day while on holiday. When your body gets used to feeding off all that sugar, you'll probably have to go through the whole withdrawal process all over again, which is not what you want. If that happens, it happens, but it's easier for you if it doesn't.

Ian Marber believes that a large part of our love for all things sweet comes down to habit and the fact that most of us indulge ourselves so often.

'Of course there is a biochemical drive to eat sweet things, which we've already discussed,' he says, 'but I think a large part of our desire for sugar comes about from habit. If you don't have any sugar for two weeks, then go and have a Sherbet Dib-Dab, for example, you would find it horrifying. It would feel as if you had a lot of heat in your mouth. Eating this kind of thing regularly, however, causes us to become numbed to that sensation. A period of time with no sugar will change your perception of what is sweet and what is not sweet. You stop enjoying it as you used to.'

Ian saying this made me think of the feeling I had the first time I drank alcohol. Do you remember how you felt? I distinctly remember stealing a sip of someone's beer at my dad's rowing club when I was very young. It tasted vile. I couldn't fathom how people would go through life ordering this stuff and drinking it in such big glasses. I felt sure it would never be for me. Yet fast forward ten years, and there I was. Likewise, when Jane gave up Diet Coke earlier this year and then tasted it again a few weeks later, she found it disgusting and wondered how on earth she ever used to drink so many cans of the stuff. Had she continued having cans, she has no doubt she soon would have become accustomed to the taste and extreme fizziness and begun to enjoy it again.

It's important to remember too, that making a new habit is a lot easier than breaking an old one. As Julia Layton writes in a piece on Howstuffworks.com (a link to which can be found in the sources section at the back of this book), research has shown that while the behavioural pathways that are formed in your brain over years of repeated actions can weaken without use, they never disappear. This means, infuriatingly, they can be 'reactivated' very easily – if you've ever tried to quit smoking, you already know this. 'You can go a year without a cigarette,' she writes, 'and then give in one time and bam! The habit comes right back.'

'Habits or cravings are bigger than the actual thing you desire', says Ian. 'Imagine if you had a friend who was chaotic with money. In her twenties she went overdrawn, maxed out her credit cards, then had to go to her parents for help. Her parents say, "we'll help you out, but I hope you've learnt your lesson", to which she replies she has. But then she does it again. And again. And again. You would possibly surmise that this person has an issue that's not about money, maybe it's an issue about entitlement, about adulthood, responsibility... If you are constantly borrowing from your mum and dad, you could argue that you want to stay rooted to them, and want to stay dependent on them for some reason. Likewise with food, eating what you want and gaining a lot of weight, then losing it, then gaining it again is almost a form of punishment and reward and keeps people trapped in a chaotic state and rooted to their original issue, which is probably little to do with food. What we eat has become a big issue that is so multi-faceted, it has very little to do with biochemistry, although we want it to be.'

So, how can you escape from this trap? Well, as making new habits are easier than breaking old ones, the easiest thing is to try and form what's called a 'parallel pattern', which you can employ whenever you feel the urge coming on. The key to this process is to know what sets you off. If you know you reach for chocolate or sweet things at 4 p.m., make sure you have some nuts or hummus and veggies handy to snack on. If you're an emotional eater and a bar of chocolate is one of the crutches you rely upon to blast away the stresses of a bad day, try introducing exercise to help you blow off some steam instead. If I had read this two years ago I would have rolled my eyes at the very suggestion, thinking 'exercise is in no way the same as having a chocolate bar! Exercise involves effort and eating a chocolate bar does not.' But exercise really can take the place of your treats and, if you keep it up for a couple of weeks, these parallel patterns will become your normal. Rather than indulging the old pattern of chocolate, which triggers your feelings for sweets when you feel stressed or bored or whatever, the gym urge will get triggered instead.

In fact, there's a growing school of thought that believes that falling off the wagon is actually a good thing when it comes to trying to give up the things we're dependent upon. I first read about this idea in a piece called 'The New Quitter', written by journalist Kat McGowan in the American magazine *Psychology Today* back in the summer of 2010. In it, the author said this: 'The dirty little secret about addictions is that relapsing is the rule, not the exception'. They went on to state that although there were over 48 million ex-smokers in the USA at the time the piece was written (which is two million more than the 46 million people quoted as current smokers), between 60 and 90 per cent of people trying to quit have a cigarette within a year of them first giving up. About 80 per cent of alcoholics seeking treatment drink again at least once. In short, the article says;

'when it comes to major behavioural changes – anything from losing weight to quitting hard drugs – few people do it perfectly the first time. For most, it's a long and winding road.'

This new 'psychology of addiction' the piece says, 'recognises that relapse is distressingly common [and] also that it can be just a stumble on the road to recovery.' In fact, it says 'if handled the right way, a relapse can actually open the door to lasting success.'

Also quoted in the feature is an eminent psychologist Dr G. Alan Marlatt, a professor, expert and author of *Relapse Prevention*, then working at the University of Washington in Seattle, who sadly died in 2011.

Dr Marlatt believed that there are two types of relapses, a lapse and a full relapse and that a lapse should be treated as a warning sign, rather than a complete failure.

'One of his early insights was that black-and-white thinking can turn a minor lapse into a major one,' Kat McGowan writes. 'After a small slip, many people throw in the towel. A new ex-smoker has a couple of drags of a friend's cigarette, bums another, and then buys a pack, figuring she's already negated all her progress. This "abstinence-violation effect," as Marlatt named it, is the belief that anything less than perfection is total failure. It leads the quitter to conclude he just doesn't have the willpower to succeed.

'Marlatt encourages the backslider to see lapses as errors rather than defeats. Instead of stewing in guilt, the quitter should think analytically about how it occurred, dissecting the circumstances. What was he feeling? What happened earlier that day? Who was around? "We try to make it a learning process," says Marlatt. "We say: 'Hey, you fell off the wagon. How would you handle it differently next time?'" With this mentality, a recovering addict can learn to identify the situations that are likely to push him into a relapse. He can embrace the possibility of failure and see the broader horizon of change beyond it.'

In other words, if you crack and drink a White Russian cocktail through a straw at 3 p.m. in the afternoon, then follow it with a glass of red wine and a bucket of chips and mayonnaise, as I told you I did in Chapter Six, it's not the end of the world. Just keep it in perspective, see it as an event in your past and move on, rather than dwelling on it and thinking you've somehow 'ruined' everything you've been working towards.

Kat's piece goes on to explain that while a lapse doesn't necessarily mean the end, it's better to develop 'coping' strategies that help to steer you away from this in the first place.

'People who use some kind of coping technique in response to an urge are 25 times more likely to resist the temptation than those who try to just gut it out,' she wrote.

Here are some strategies she quotes in her piece:

Planning

Come up with a scheme to counteract or avoid your habit and foresee situations that could potentially prove difficult for you. Whether that's not going into the newsagent where you normally buy your chocolate bars, ordering your food online rather than browsing the supermarket aisles or choosing a restaurant that offers an array of things that are low sugar if you're going out for dinner.

Cognitive tricks or so-called 'urge surfing'

When you feel a craving, 'mentally detach yourself from the urge by watching how your desire builds then recedes'.

Developing meaningful life goals

Swap the cocktail for feeling comfortable in your bikini on the beach this summer. Skip the dessert so you can get fitter and start to enjoy outside activities.

The third point, above, taps in to what Amanda Hills has to say on the psychology of abstinence. I asked her if there were steps you can take to help your mind keep your body on track.

'The secret to abstinence is motivation,' she says. 'If someone implements a lifestyle change, such as giving up sugar, and it begins to make them look better, feel better, to act better or be better in some way, then it has its own impetus. With sugar, when you start feeling you have more energy and you see you're losing weight, that your skin and eyes become clearer, that your hair looks shinier, you feel less stressed and your moods improve, you no longer feel such an acute desire for "treat" food. We know human beings are suckers for reward, but those changes are reward enough. You're motivated by not wanting to go back to the way you were before. If you do lapse and you go back to your old ways – perhaps you go out for cocktails with friends and indulge in too many, you wake up in the morning and think "*yuk*". It reinforces the idea that you made the right choice when you gave up and you've effectively swapped your old reward for a new one.'

This is something I can relate to. Although I'm not a hardcore gym-goer, exercise, or what I call 'actively relaxing' – yoga, pilates, swimming – has now become an important element of my life. Whereas before I would wake up tired and lie in bed until as late as I possibly could to make it to work on time (well, more or less on time), these days I don't mind getting up early in the morning. I often plan my day to start with a bit of exercise fairly early on – whether that's going to the gym before heading into the office or doing a yoga video from YouTube in the dining room before eating my breakfast. I know it sounds disgustingly wholesome, but it's actually kind of enjoyable. Of course, sometimes I really don't feel like dragging myself out from beneath the covers, but once I am up and moving it's fine. Best of all it's one hour that I know will make me feel good for the rest of the day.

And it's a means to an end. Making a commitment to doing something first thing in the morning certainly puts paid to any hankering for those late-night drinking sessions I used to get up to (not that I ever really want to do that any more).

If you're lacking in willpower or aren't particularly a morning person, try roping someone else in to do it with you. I often arrange to meet someone else to exercise with – either I'm going to the Bodyism gym where one of the trainers will help me through a workout, or I'm driving eight miles or so to west London to see Holly Pannett for a personal training session, or I'll have arranged to meet my friend Ruth for an early morning cycle class or my friend Sam for a jog around the park. There's nothing like knowing someone else has hauled themselves out of bed to meet you to guilt you into getting into your gym kit.

Ultimately, when it comes to staying the distance it's important to remember that you are in charge of your own success or failure, and the person who has the most to gain from you succeeding at extracting that sweet tooth of yours, is you.

Chapter Ten

LOW SUGAR
AND THE FUTURE

The other night over a work dinner, a lady I've never met before asked me how old I was. I told her I was 35. She appeared shocked, turned to our neighbour and said 'Nicole could be ten years younger. Her skin is amazing!' Of course, a lot of this is bluster and the restaurant was also pretty dark, which is always more forgiving. I don't think I look much younger than I am, but nevertheless, she mentioned my skin. I was beyond chuffed. Someone commenting positively on my skin is something that never would have happened to me two years ago. People never used to mention my skin, because it was pretty bad – red, inflamed and congested.

In 2012, I was an overweight, unhappy, stressed-out moody woman, with spots and bad habits. I was exhausted and pretty often ill. I didn't really realise I was doing this to myself because of what I ate. In fact, I always thought it was something else that was to blame for my various malaises; often it was my job, sometimes getting over a relationship breakdown, then there was my heart condition or something else that couldn't completely be pinned on me. There was no way, I reasoned, that it was me that was causing all of these negative elements of my life. What's more, there was little I could do to remedy them. What could I do about my love life? My heart condition was something that doctors took care of, not something I could control. And I needed to work to pay my mortgage. My life overwhelmed me. I was constantly worried and anxious, fearful, on the back foot. I didn't feel in control of myself, let alone anything else.

But, as you know, one day I just woke up and took responsibility for my life. I realised that the only person that could change most of those things was me. It was pointless my going around making out there was nothing that could be done about my weight. Of course there was. And my weight was what bothered me the most. Not only for vanity reasons, although I am probably vainer than I would care to admit, but because I didn't want to be unhealthy. We all know carrying excess weight is not good for us and I already had a heart condition. Sure, carrying a couple of extra pounds isn't the end of the world, but our national obesity problem is only growing, and the bigger it grows, the more strain it puts on the already overloaded National Health Service.

So, quite simply, I took a short, hard look at what I ate, identified the problem and decided to fix it. I succeeded, because I really wanted to. I was determined not to fail in this because I had read that cutting back on sugar was a sustainable long-term way to improve your health and that was what I wanted. I'm not a nutritionist or an expert in any way, I didn't want to do something that was hard to follow or meant that I couldn't go out to dinner or lunch. I also did not want to go on a diet that focuses only on your waistline in a short-term, unsustainable way. I just hoped giving up sugar would work for me.

It did. The results were visible in a matter of days. After my eyes became bright and glittery, my waistline started to shrink. My taste buds and sense of smell went into overdrive, my skin cleared up. You know what happened, you've read the book.

If you eat a lot of sugar, as I used to, I can pretty much guarantee you will feel like a different person if you give it up. You will feel brighter and lighter in a matter of weeks. I've talked about weight a lot in this book, which is ironic because until two years ago I hardly talked about it at all. I never mentioned it to boyfriends, or friends in general, because I thought there was nothing more boring than someone who doesn't like their appearance. Besides, I was never hugely fat. At most I was a size 16, which is pretty easy to carry off when you are 5′10″, as I am. And I put on an outwardly confident façade that I never ever let drop – not even when I lived with people for years. I fooled everybody, except for my family and myself.

Cutting out most forms of sugar has meant my whole life has changed. I'm still the same person, but a different version of her. I'm neither better nor worse, but I'm certainly altered. And I am much happier.

I know this is going to read like a recruiting poster for some weird cult, but do you want to change any of the things I mentioned above? Are you sick of feeling ill and tired, of having bad skin and hormonal problems? Perhaps you want to lose some weight that's proving tough to shift? If you have a diet similar to my old one, in other words high-sugar cereals and a juice for breakfast, a lunch of either bread or rice and then a dinner of pasta or similar – not forgetting a couple of sweet snacks throughout the day – then you know what you have to do.

But there is no miracle cure. Just stick with it. Make foods from scratch, eat more protein. Fall in love with eggs and all the delicious things you can do with them. Go wild in the aisles and discover new things. What in the world are buckwheat groats and what do they taste like? Who even knew cocoa nibs existed? What is almond butter like, or unsweetened peanut butter for that matter? There are emerald green rich-buttery tasting queen olives the size of walnuts that will set your tastebuds aquiver and black beans that can be mashed up to make cakes. See your new regime as an opportunity, not a chore.

It's not all great news. Going low sugar can be expensive. Ready meals and convenience foods are, on the whole, cheap, especially if you are cooking for one. But low-sugar living doesn't have to be extortionate. Holly's recipe for the tarka dahl-ing (see page 200) costs under £7 to make and it serves four. That's either dinner for a group of you, or dinner and two lunches for you. If you can't afford organic meat, buy free range. If you can't afford free range, buy what you can afford. Do your best. No one's going to judge you.

Talking of which, friendships. Two years on, how have mine faired? On the whole, very well. Many of my friends are still surprised that I don't eat much sugar. One of the most common questions I get asked by some of my nearest and dearest is 'are you *still* not eating sugar?' whenever we go out for dinner and I swerve the first glass of wine or avoid the basket of scrumptious white bread. But these days it's almost always followed by 'I can't believe it, you've done so well,' or 'I wish I could do it'.

The great thing is growing numbers of people are doing it. Huge campaigns from prominent national newspapers have drawn the issue of sugar to our attention. Indeed, in spring, the *Daily Mail* gave away a free handbag-sized guide to the amounts of sugar in foods to help shoppers make healthier low-sugar choices in the aisles. It feels as if the nation is waking up to how much unnecessary sweetness is being added to lots of the things we all buy, and we're shocked.

Not so long ago, of course, it would have been impossible to imagine a time when people couldn't smoke in pubs or restaurants. Back in the days when commuters used to light up on the underground on their way into work, or sit in the 'smoking section' of an airplane to go on holiday, puffing away was seen as a socially acceptable pastime, that was well beyond the meddling reach of governments, regulators or lawmakers. Indeed, even when I got my first job on a newspaper in 2003, journalists used to be allowed to light up at their desk after 6 p.m. (before that it was only allowed in the stairwell, which was a rather unfortunate welcome for us breathless individuals who favoured climbing the five flights up to the office rather than taking the lift). It was deemed a Briton's right to pretty much do as they pleased when it came to fags. Those who complained about it were lambasted as busy bodies who wanted to curtail other people's civil liberties; neurotic health-freaks who needed to mind their own business. In spite of the clear and proven health risks to both smokers and those breathing in second-hand smoke, lawmakers shied away from imposing restrictions on smoking for a long time.

Then, in 2007, the Government put the smoking ban into place in England. The benefits of such action did not take long to show up. It triggered the biggest fall in the habit ever seen in the country. Since its inception, hospitals have seen significant reductions in the numbers of people being admitted with heart and asthma attacks.

These days we no longer cherish our smoke-free bars and eateries – it's normal. Nor do we want to be able to smoke in a shopping mall, for instance. We don't think about the days that we used to come home from a night out and put our clothes straight into the washing machine because they smelled too strongly of fags to wear again. It doesn't occur to us anymore that a taxi driver could take you to your destination while puffing away on a cigarette, regardless of whether you liked it or not.

A few years ago, I went to visit my friends Guy and Toby who live in Verbier and run their own ski school called Performance Verbier. It's a heavenly mountainside village, 1500 metres above sea level up in the Swiss Alps. Being at altitude means the air is crisp and fresh. In the winter it's cold and invigorating. That is, until you go inside where people were chugging away on fags like they were going out of fashion – which they were. My eyes burned. The air was such a fug, I felt headachy, congested and hungover after a couple of drinks. Opening the door to my room the next evening after a day on the ski slopes (and I do, literally spend most of the day on the slopes trying to get up after falling over), there was a pungent smell of tobacco smoke emanating from the chair in the corner of the room. It was where I had left the clothes I had been wearing the night before.

Despite being one of the last bastions to allow it, Switzerland has also now banned smoking. It's now completely accepted even among my few friends who do still smoke, that it needed to be regulated for the good of the general population.

Fast forward to 2015, and is it possible that the sale of sugar will eventually become regulated in the way that tobacco is? I've already talked about the World Health Organization (WHO) recommendation that we all halve the amount of sugar we consume. That would mean we would receive just 5 per cent of our daily energy intake from sugar. To make it easier to picture, that equates to about 6 level teaspoons of the white stuff per day. The levels will be lower for children.

At this moment in time – March 2014 – a quick internet search of the phrase 'sugar is the new tobacco' (using those quote marks means you search for the exact phrase rather than just the individual words) gets 459,000 results. I wager if you do it now – whenever you are reading this – there will be many more.

There are plenty of conspiracy theorists out there who spout their theories that Western governments allow the wholesale pollution of our foods with sugar because it makes the population happier and therefore easier to control (yup, pretty nuts). But recent years have seen several well-known authorities on sugar come out and say they believe sugar is the equivalent of tobacco for children. They have often been derided by the establishment as misguided scaremongers.

Take paediatric endocrinologist Professor Robert Lustig from the University of California, who has been criticised by some elements of the medical establishment and the food manufacturing industry. Professor Lustig has become the pin-up boy of the anti-sugar movement. His book *Fat Chance* generated headlines around the world when it was published at the end of 2012 and his must-watch 90-minute lecture 'The Bitter Truth' has had over 4.5 million views on YouTube.

Yet despite popular acclaim, many in the food and medical establishment vehemently disagree with his hypothesis that sugar doesn't just make you fat and rot your teeth, but it causes several chronic and very common illnesses, including heart disease, cancer, Alzheimer's and diabetes. They also don't agree that it's addictive and that, in its fructose form, it suppresses the hormone leptin, which tells you when you're full, causing you to eat too much without realising.

While Professor Lustig is the most famous, he was by no means the first sugar sceptic. The sources section of this book links to a fascinating piece in the *Telegraph* on British professor John Yudkin, who wrote a book called *Pure, White and Deadly* in 1972 that issued what are now being deemed 'prophetic' warnings about the dangers of eating lots of sweet things. His theory was that it wasn't fat that was making us fat and ill, but sugar. This flew in the face of the new nutritional advice at the time that told everyone to cut fat out of their diets and instead, eat low-fat products (many of which had often been flavoured with sugar). Saying Yudkin's work was unpopular puts it mildly. He became the subject of an organised campaign by the food industry to discredit him.

Publishing *Pure, White and Deadly* effectively ended Yudkin's career. It has, however, recently been republished with a foreword by Professor Lustig.

Because, although Professor Yudkin is no longer alive to see it, the tide is finally turning against sugar. People are increasingly realising that, in Professor Lustig's words, 'it ain't the fat, people. It ain't the fat'.

In March 2014, Francesco Branca, Director for Nutrition for Health and Development at the WHO, told the *Daily Mail* newspaper that sugar and other risk factors are often linked to obesity which affects half a billion people in the world and it is set to become the new tobacco in terms of public health action. Weight gain, particularly in children, can be linked to the consumption of sugar sweetened beverages. She advised that drinks such as soda can often exceed a child's daily limit of sugar and should be approached with care.

The WHO advice is by no means set in stone – there are still panels and committees of experts that need to get behind these new advisories. But in the same month, *The Times* newspaper reported that Britain's Chief Medical Officer Dame Sally Davies had said people did not realise that fruit juices, smoothies and fizzy drinks were 'highly calorific', and should be taken in moderation.

Dame Davies feels sure that new research will show that sugar is addictive and is urging the government to regulate the food industry saying 'I think with the science we will find sugar is addictive... We need a big education [programme] and may need to move to some form of sugar tax.' This tax would raise money to help deal with the knock-on health effects of our national obesity crisis. Indeed, it's been reported that research by Oxford and Reading universities found that a tax of 20 per cent would cut the number of obese people in this country by 180,000.

So, there you have it. The idea of significantly cutting back on our sugar intake has gone mainstream. It's no longer solely the preserve of woo-woo health freaks and nutritionists but is being recommended by the country's most important doctor, and in all probability, the British government too before long.

The subject of sugar in our foods also looks set to become a party political issue in the run-up to the 2015 general election. The Labour party is already considering imposing a maximum limit for sugar, salt and fat in products aimed at children while the Conservatives have claimed that they would work with the food industry in order that it brings down the levels of sugar voluntarily, as has been done with salt. There have, of course, already been cries of 'nanny state' meddling from some politicians.

I spoke to Professor Graham MacGregor, who is a cardiologist and the chairman of Action on Sugar, a group of 18 specialists concerned with sugar and its effects on our health. Their aim is to work with both the food industry and the Government to bring about a reduction in the amount of sugar in our processed foods. They have already achieved this with levels of salt, through their group Consensus Action on Salt and Health.

'What we are trying to do is to stop people from suffering or dying prematurely – particularly from cardiovascular disease and cancer,' Professor MacGregor says. 'The major causes of cardiovascular disease and cancer are diet and smoking. The three factors that are important in diet are firstly, salt, because that puts up your blood pressure – and high blood pressure is the biggest killer in the world by far. Secondly, saturated fat which puts up our cholesterol and is a very big source of calories – one tablespoon of olive oil is the equivalent of four apples in terms of calories. Then lastly, there's added sugar.

'Nobody ever put salt on their meals until a few thousand years ago and it's a similar thing with sugar. We didn't add it to things until it was made cheap by slave labour a few hundred years ago. Sugar is an unnecessary source of calories in our diet. We don't notice we are eating it and if we do eat it, we don't feel satiated by it. Therefore, it's a problem in causing obesity – and therefore indirectly diabetes – not to mention tooth decay.

'The aim of our action group is to do what we did

with salt – we got the food industry to slowly take salt out of their foods. The quantities of salt you find in the foods you buy from the supermarket have now come down by approximately 30 per cent.

'Nobody's realised. Food manufacturers could do the same for sugar, they could just slowly take it out without anybody realising. From a public health point of view, that would be brilliant because it affects everybody in the population. You're buying the same food but eating less.

'The public can't detect these subtle changes and we don't go around saying "these products have got less salt in" because people won't buy it. It's slightly different with sugar because people are more aware of sugar and more keen to cut it out of their diet, but we would rather manufacturers just did it unobtrusively without telling anyone.

'The food industry could take out 10 per cent of all the sugar in sweetened soft drinks tomorrow and in a year's time they could do another 10 per cent, and another 10 per cent the year after that so in three years you have a 30 per cent reduction in sugar in soft drinks worldwide. That would have a huge effect on calorie intake from a pubic health perspective.'

So, what does Professor MacGregor think we should do?

'Clearly we need to reduce our calorie intake, we need to reduce our salt intake and our saturated fat intake. I never eat sugar, I don't enjoy it. If you don't eat something, you stop liking the taste of it. You can't get rid of the food industry – unfortunately, however much we'd like to – they're too powerful. Therefore you have to get them to try and modify the appalling foods they're selling by making them more healthy – that's our aim.'

Another aim needs to be for big food companies to demystify what is put into their products. Most people would have no idea that sugar is added to salad dressings, soups, pasta sauces and the like. The information has been confusing for too long. Even the NHS appears to offer confusing, irresponsible advice. As of March 2014, the NHS's own Live Well website has an information page called 'A Balanced Diet', which issues the following laughable advice about cutting back on sugar: 'Have a currant bun as a snack instead of a pastry.' I think most of us would agree a currant bun, with its sticky sweet glaze, its white flour and sugary dried fruit, is hardly a healthy alternative to anything.

So, let's recap what we're talking about when we talk about sugar. These WHO guidelines mostly focus on added sugars in the ready-made products we buy, the so-called 'empty calories'. These are the worst kind of sugars, the ones that are added to our food and drinks, the ones many of us don't really know we're eating. These are the sugars that are secreted in our ready meals, our shop-bought biscuits and cakes, our fizzy drinks, some of our processed meats, crisps, sauces, breads, muesli bars, on-the-go breakfast cereals (such as flavoured instant porridge), salad dressings, coleslaws and soups. The sugars in our low-fat or fat-free diet products such as frozen yoghurt, cereals, flavoured yoghurts, even branded products from specialist weight-loss companies like Slim Fast whose shakes in a can contain as much as 5½ teaspoons of sugar. Remember, you can often find these ingredients by looking for things that end in '–ose' or 'syrup' in an ingredients list on a product. The stuff we add to our foods ourselves also counts in our added sugar intake, but the good thing about this is we know how much we are adding so it's easier to cut back. Nowadays it is considered slightly old fashioned to add white sugar to your porridge in the morning, but if you do, that's one thing you can cut back on easily. Brown or unrefined sugars are pretty similar to white sugars but some have just been through less processing at the factory. They cause the body to react in the exact same way that white sugar does. Try using ground cinnamon on top of things or in your drinks instead.

Where things start to get confusing is with honey, agave, maple syrup and the like. They're often less refined, but are they just as bad as sugar? I got into an animated debate about this over a recent breakfast with a group of health-industry professionals and journalists who were interested in the low-sugar movement. Many people believe it is okay to use agave, honey and maple syrup on their foods because it was in some way better than sugar. I proclaimed it was not much better than sugar and this is why.

Although this simplifies things slightly, our bodies will react to maple syrup, honey and agave in much same way as they will react to any other sweet thing we ingest. While many of these products are less refined than granulated sugars (some have the words 'raw' or 'unrefined' written on their label), many aren't and, even so, both forms still cause blood sugar spikes in the same way that granulated sugars do. Granted, the more natural sugars do contain some trace minerals – honey for example is a natural antiseptic and contains niacin, riboflavin, thiamine and vitamin B6, but those minerals only make up about 2 per cent of honey's total content so it's not as healthy as some people make out. When you compare that 2 per cent to the 55 per cent of fructose that honey's made of (you'll remember that fructose is the sugar processed directly by the liver, which eaten in excess, contributes to obesity and heart problems), 2 per cent is really no great shakes. In discussions about honey, and the like, the words 'natural' and 'better for you' usually get bandied about a lot. The only way these alternative sugars are 'better' is in our minds because we imbue them with a sense of somehow being more natural than granulated white sugar. Granulated sugar, of course, comes from sugar beet and sugar cane, so it's also 'natural'. My advice is, if you can, hugely limit your intake of honey, agave and maple syrup if you are trying to cut out sugar. Not only do they cause blood sugar spikes, They also maintain your palette's taste for sweet things. I try not to eat them at all unless I can't avoid it or I'm having a treat or making a dessert for people coming around for dinner.

Then, there are the sugars contained in natural foods that we don't really want. In their new recommendations, the WHO has said that people should continue eating whole fruit because what it provides in terms of sugar is more than offset by its abundant vitamins, minerals and fibre. You all know, however, that I only eat fruit very occasionally. This admission often provokes scorn and incredulity when I tell people, but I'm not afflicted with scurvy and haven't had a cold since I ditched fruit so I must be doing something right. In fact, it's quite common for lots of people who are low sugar not to eat fruit – several eminent specialists I have interviewed both for this book and for other articles on the subject also don't.

'One type of sugar being somehow "better" than another type is a psychological issue, in this country and the United States,' says Ian Marber. 'When we have an inferior alternative to something, we elevate the slightly superior. For example, when you could have had a meringue, but instead you only have strawberries, you feel quite saintly. But the truth of the matter is, your strawberries choice isn't great either, it's just better than the meringue. It's like having your car stopped by the police after having half a bottle of wine and saying "but I could have had two bottles". You're still over the limit. Fructose [fruit sugar, which is both naturally occurring and added to things] gets processed by the liver and when you eat too much of it, it prompts the liver to start producing glucose through a process called gluconeogenesis – put simply, new glucose formation. Although fructose doesn't affect glucose levels in the blood directly, it's only one step removed. The result is more or less the same.'

Of course, becoming low sugar is about becoming more healthy, not less, and it's important to still get vitamins, minerals, and fibre from fresh produce. You should not hugely lower your intake of fruit without significantly increasing the number of vegetables and what I call low-sugar fruits – namely dark berries (blackberries, blueberries, raspberries) that you eat. This is imperative. And when it comes to sugar, all fruits are not created equal. Dark berries do not have as big an effect on our blood sugar levels as fruits like pineapples, peaches, bananas, apples and pears, which are some of the worst offenders when it comes to creating blood sugar spikes. If cutting out fruit altogether sounds too difficult for you, just try cutting back. Eat lower sugar fruits rather than slabs of pineapple and punnets of peaches and graze on nuts at the same time. Doing so dampens down the body's response to the sugar you're taking on board (more of this on page 298).

While vegetables can also be broken down into two similar categories – the starchy and the non-starchy (the former raise your blood sugars more than the latter), I tend to eat both types of vegetable with the exception of potatoes (I've replaced them with sweet potatoes as they have a lower GI).

Talking of which, foods that turn to sugar inside your body are the last of the four different forms of sugar I've discussed. These don't necessarily taste sweet in the mouth so they're less easy to identify by taste, but if you need help, charts indicating the Glycaemic Index (GI) of various foods are readily available online or you can download an app that will help you until you get the hang of it. It's a sliding scale, and the foods that have a high GI – pasta, white rice, many forms of bread, etc. – are quickly converted to sugar when they're ingested which isn't what the body needs. To ensure long-term energy, fewer highs and lows and feeling fuller for longer, it's better to go for foods that have a low GI – brown rice, lentils and pulses and wholegrains such as quinoa, amaranth, spelt and buckwheat.

When you do eat something sweet – and the likelihood is that you will, no matter how firm your resolve – what also matters is what you eat it with. We know the body can deal with sugar best when it's accompanied by protein and fat, so having blueberries with some nuts on your porridge helps slow the absorption of the sugar into your body and minimises blood sugar spikes and crashes. This is also why it's better not to eat sweet things on an empty stomach.

As I've already mentioned, if this feels like too much for you to give up at once, do it gradually. Start by eliminating all added sugars – ready meals, processed foods like biscuits and cakes, muesli bars, fizzy drinks and anything you eat on the go. Artificially sweetened 'low-sugar' or 'sugar-free' products that use man-made synthetic sweeteners need to be ditched too – and don't forget honey, agave, maple syrup and any other alternative sweeteners you have been using. If you sweeten your tea or coffee, stop. Once you have conquered those things, try to cut back on the high GI foods – bread, pasta, white rice and the like. Then, when you have done with those, gradually cut back on your fruit. This process doesn't have to be drastic; you can do it over a period of weeks if you need to. The important thing is that you do it. Your body will thank you for it.

'Clients who eat a lot of sugar are always tired' says Lee Mullins of Bodyism. 'They're lacking in energy. While they're not always overweight – some people can get away with eating lots of sugar without storing lots of fat – this doesn't mean what is going on inside their bodies is going to be good. Sugar creates an environment for inflammation inside the body and inflammation has been linked to diseases. Bodyism's founder James Duigan says "life is short, but it's also really long". I know that sounds funny, but what we mean by that is that we'll have about 80 years to spend on this planet. Eighty years is a long time to spend tired or feeling unwell, so it pays to start looking after your body now.'

We all know that stopping eating sugar is one thing we can do for our bodies and minds that will lead to almost instantaneous improvements. But what should you do to help your face?

'Today's young women will age worse than older women do now,' says Mica Engel, the aesthetic doctor I mentioned earlier. 'Not only because of smoking or sun damage – although these play key parts – a lot of it is because we have been much more exposed to higher levels of sugar than any of the previous generations who were not raised on foods containing things like high fructose corn syrup.

'There is sugar in much of the things we eat. Most processed food is just full of junk. The older generation had a much better diet and the effects of what we eat are shown on our faces. We eat fast food, live fast lives, everything has to be easy. It's not good for our bodies or our skin.

'I'm not only a cosmetic doctor, I was an A&E doctor at home in Brazil and did a postgraduate qualification in preventative medicine. I'm very interested in how to not get sick on a microscopic molecular level. There is lots of research that shows calorie restriction prolongs life because it reduces glycation [the inflammatory process whereby excess sugar molecules bind themselves to fats and proteins in your body, which leads to the skin's protein fibres becoming brittle and stiff and skin appearing aged]. Minimising inflammation like this is not only important for your skin, it's really important for your health as well.'

Changing your diet will, of course, have huge benefits for your skin – and plenty more besides. But rectifying the damage done by the foods we eat is sure to be the Next Big Thing in skincare. Well-regarded clinical skincare brand SkinCeuticals was among the first to bring out a range specifically aimed at dulled, grey and prematurely aged glycated skins, which has fared well in independent clinical testing done over a three-month period. Their A.G.E. Interrupter (Advanced Glycation End-products) cream has been designed to 'reverse the erosion of elasticity and firmness caused by Advanced Glycation End-products'. This is what it says on the back of the jar 'Glycation occurs when excess sugar molecules stick to collagen and elastin fibres, binding to them and causing chemical reactions called A.G.E… These reactions reduce the fibres' regenerative ability, leading to severe wrinkling of the skin.'

Sounds good, but at £143 for a jar (which should last about three months), you'd expect it to be. If that's beyond your price range, take heart from this from Mica.

'Acne can be vastly improved by changing your diet,' she says. 'In fact, you can completely restructure your skin by not eating inflammatories like sugar. It has a massive effect.'

And it does, I am proof of that. Now, two years on, I realise I have become something of an evangelist for not eating as much sugar, but let's get one thing straight. It's not the cure-all. From time to time I still get spots, I have one of the little blighters right now just in the middle of my chin. I'm also not a skinny beanpole, I'm a size 12 or so, maybe a 10 in some things. But I am a world away from where I was before.

Last night I lay in bed wondering what my life would be like if I still ate and drank in the same way that I used to. What would I look like? How would I have coped with breaking up with Barry, leaving my job, moving house? Would I still be spending inordinate amounts of my money on a skincare routine that didn't really come close to addressing the issues that were causing my problems in the first place? Would I still be rushing to the gym to pound a treadmill, rewarding myself with a fruit yoghurt or a smoothie straight afterwards, then wondering why I wasn't losing any weight? Could I ever have got over all of those extreme emotional highs and lows I used to feel, or would I just have found something else to blame?

I urge you to give living low sugar a try. See how you feel. You know it's going to be tough at times, but you have the knowledge to do it and you're well prepared.

In the beginning it's going to take more effort to track down some of the weirder things that you'll use to supplement your diet (although things like quinoa and coconut oil are already being sold in savvy supermarkets like Sainsbury's that are cottoning on to all things healthy), but you know it's worth it, for your heart, your mind and your looks.

I can't stress enough how unlikely the last two years of my life have been. Had anyone told me in 2012 that I would be writing a book on how to live healthily I would have laughed in their face. People say going low sugar is hard, and it is, for a short while. But if I can do it – me, the girl who spent Saturdays hiding in the passport photo booth in Woolworths eating pick-n-mix without paying; the girl who ate those chalky Lucozade tablets as sweets after having a McDonald's milkshake most Saturdays as a teenager; the girl who reached for a chocolate biscuit from bed before she opened her eyes in her halls of residence... If I can do this, anyone can.

SOURCES

INTRODUCTION:

Sources for the quantities of sugar in our daily foods comes from the Daily Mail's 'How Much Sugar Is In Your Food' guide given away with the paper in February 2014

Obesity nearly tripled in UK since 1980:

NHS UK, 'Obesity and its effects', http://www.health4work.nhs.uk/blog/2012/02/obesity-and-its-effects/ <2 February 2012 >

NHS guidelines on how much sugar is acceptable:

NHS UK, 'How much sugar is good for me?', 'http://www.nhs.uk/chq/pages/1139.aspx?categoryid=51&subcategoryid=167 <17 May 2013>

NHS estimate that we eat around 700g of sugar per week:

NHS UK, 'How to cut down on sugar in your own diet',

http://www.nhs.uk/Livewell/Goodfood/Pages/How-to-cut-down-on-sugar-in-your-diet.aspx <28 January 2014>

Britons are buying less bags of sugar:

William Leith, 'The bitter truth about sugar', http://www.telegraph.co.uk/health/dietandfitness/9160114/The-bitter-truth-about-sugar.html <27 March 2012>

Sugar consumption has more than tripled in the past 50 years:

Robert H. Lustig, Laura A. Schmidt and Claire D. Brindis, 'The Toxic Truth about Sugar', *Nature*, vol. 482, 2012, pp.27-29.

CHAPTER ONE:

Britons eat a staggering 24lbs of chocolate on average per year:

CNN, 'Who consumes the most chocolate?', http://thecnnfreedomproject.blogs.cnn.com/2012/01/17/who-consumes-the-most-chocolate/ <17 January 2012>

Neotame 7000-13000 times sweeter than sugar:

Harvard Health Publications, 'Are artificial sweeteners safe?',

http://www.health.harvard.edu/healthbeat/HEALTHbeat_033005.htm

CHAPTER TWO:

Brain scans showing food addiction:

Science Daily, 'New brain imaging study provides support for the notion of food addiction', http://www.sciencedaily.com/releases/2013/06/130626153922.htm <26 June 2013>

History of sugar:

Anne Gibson, 'How we became addicted to sugar', BBC History, http://www.bbc.co.uk/history/0/20311399 <26 November 2012>

Wikipedia, 'History of sugar', http://en.wikipedia.org/wiki/History_of_sugar

Rachel Nuwer, 'Blame Napoleon for Our Addiction to Sugar',

http://www.smithsonianmag.com/smart-news/blame-napoleon-for-our-addiction-to-sugar-152096743/?no-ist <4 December 2012>

'White Gold':

Sugar Nutrition UK, 'History of sugar', http://www.sugarnutrition.org.uk/history-of-sugar.aspx

2013 national diet and nutrition survey:

Rosie Boycott, 'We're all sugar junkies now', http://www.dailymail.co.uk/health/article-2420713/Were-sugar-junkies-Britons-wolf-unimaginable-160-teaspoons-week--worse-news-It-really-IS-addictive.html <14 September 2013>

Sugars in fruit and dried fruit:

Loren Cordain, 'Fruits and sugars: Sugar content of fruit', http://thepaleodiet.com/fruits-and-sugars/

Food for the brain interview with Deborah Colson on the link between sugar and stress:

Nicole Mowbray, 'The real reason you feel stressed… SUGAR',
http://www.*dailymail*.co.uk/femail/article-2399351/SUGAR-real-reason-feel-stressed-Learn-CAN-break-habit.html <21 August 2013>

CHAPTER 3:
Sweet tooth may be genetic:
Andy Bloxham, 'Scientists discover sweet tooth gene', http://www.*telegraph*.co.uk/news/1954199/Scientists-discover-sweet-tooth-gene.html <14 May 2008>
The World Health Organisation considers reducing sugar RDAs:
Kate Mansey and Jon Ungoed-Thomas, 'Sweet but deadly', http://www.*thesundaytimes*.co.uk/sto/news/uk_news/Health/Sugar/article1357404.ece<29 December 2013>
Sugar Nutrition UK and Associated British Foods:
Jon Ungoed-Thomas, 'Sweet but deadly', http://www.*thesundaytimes*.co.uk/sto/news/uk_news/Health/Sugar/article1357404.ece<29 December 2013>

CHAPTER 4:
Research from Leiden University and Unilever's Research and Development department into high blood sugar levels causing premature skin ageing:
Unilever, 'High blood sugar levels make you look older, new research suggests', http://www.*unilever*.com/mediacentre/pressreleases/2011/Highbloodsugarlevels-makeyoulookoldernewresearchsuggests.aspx <1 December 2011>
Interview with Victoria Beckham's dermatologist:
Mail Online, 'Health notes: Posh 'fixed her face with diet – not botox', http://www.*dailymail*.co.uk/health/article-2565523/Health-Notes-Posh-fixed-face-diet-not-botox-says-dermatologist.html <22 February 2014>

CHAPTER 5:
Harvard School of Public Health findings on artificial sweeteners:
Harvard School of Public Health, 'Artificial Sweeteners', http://www.*hsph.harvard*.edu/nutritionsource/healthy-drinks/artificial-sweeteners/

CHAPTER 9:
Who eats the most chocolate?:
Oliver Nieburg, 'Top 20 chocolate consuming nations of 2012', http://www.*confectionerynews*.com/Markets/Interactive-Map-Top-20-chocolate-consuming-nations-of-2012 <30 July 2013>
Stages of change model:
Wikipedia, 'Transtheoretical model', http://en.*wikipedia*.org/wiki/Transtheoretical_model
On making and breaking habits:
Julia Layton, 'Is it true that if you do anything for three weeks it will become a habit?', http://science.*howstuffworks*.com/life/form-a-habit1.htm
Janet Rae-Dupree, 'Can you become a creature of new habits?', http://www.*nytimes*.com/2008/05/04/business/04unbox.html?_r&_r=0 <4 May 2008>
Cathryn M. Delude, 'Brain researchers explain why old habits die hard', http://*newsoffice*.mit.edu/2005/habit <19 October 2005>
The psychology of addiction and relapse:
Kat McGowan, 'The New Quitter', http://www.*psychologytoday*.com/articles/201007/the-new-quitter <1 July 2010>

CHAPTER 10:
The health benefits of the smoking ban:
Sarah Boseley, 'Smoking ban 'has reduced asthma and heart attacks', http://www.*theguardian*.com/society/2012/jun/29/smoking-ban-health-benefits <29 June 2012>